T0123625

Mom,
I Have Cancer

A Story of a Journey in Faith

Barbara Vigue with Gabrielle Vigue

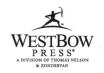

WESTBOW
P R E S S®
A DIVISION OF THOMAS NELSON
& ZONDERVAN

WestBow Press books may be ordered through booksellers or by contacting:

WestBow Press
A Division of Thomas Nelson & Zondervan
1663 Liberty Drive
Bloomington, IN 47403
www.westbowpress.com
1 (866) 928-1240

Scripture quotations marked KJV are taken from the King James Version.

Scripture quotations marked NKJV are taken from the New King James Version®. Copyright © 1982 by Thomas Nelson. Used by permission. All rights reserved.

ISBN: 978-1-9736-7708-6 (sc)
ISBN: 978-1-9736-7710-9 (hc)
ISBN: 978-1-9736-7709-3 (e)

Library of Congress Control Number: 2019915892

Print information available on the last page.

WestBow Press rev. date: 10/29/2019

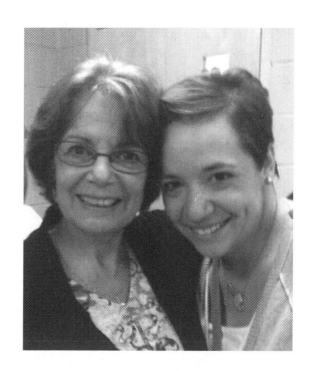

Dedicated to my daughter Gabrielle, a champion of faith who was not moved by what she saw, but by every word of God.

And

Dedicated to my loved ones, Ben, David, and Cindy who may have lost a battle, but won the war. And to all those who was now in the midst of their battle.

****

Preface

It is not my intention to write a new book on healing. Many great ones are already available. Nor is it my intention to diminish the valiant fight that many believers have fought against illness. It is only my intention to tell our journey in faith through understanding the plans and purposes of God since the beginning of time. It is my prayer that it will encourage others to stand on the unchanging Word of God for themselves.

Note: Bible references are from the King James Version. When you see [] within a Bible quote, the definition was taken from Strong's Concordance on E-Sword.com. Italic within a quotation is my emphasis added to that quotation.

Contents

CHAPTER ONE
The Journey Begins

Sometimes you can start a routine day not aware that the events of that day may change your life forever. A day like that happened for me on a Thursday morning in February. I had just finished my staff meeting at the Florida home care agency where I worked as a psychiatric nurse when I got a call from my twenty-eight-year- old daughter who lived in the Washington DC area.

She was always a strong person, but I heard the quiet quiver in her voice as she told me, "Mom, the doctors say I have cancer. Lymphoma."

I replied calmer than I felt. "Okay honey. I'll tell Dad and the reinforcements are on the way."

I hung up the phone and began to weep. Turning to another nurse, I said in unbelief, "My daughter has cancer." She grabbed me gently by the shoulders and spoke firmly to me. "You are a person of faith, Barbara." I smiled and nodded.

Now I turned to the task of calling my husband. This time it was my voice that quivered. He noticed it and admonished me, "We can't afford to allow ourselves a moment of fear or unbelief." He decided to immediately get in the car and drive the twelve-hour trip to be with our daughter. I stayed home until I could make arrangements for my elderly mom to get back to her home in Connecticut.

Bill spent three days with Gabrielle and her roommate expounding on what the Bible has to say about healing and faith.

Then I flew in to stay with her and for the next week we continued searching the scriptures for every word of God on the subject of healing and faith.

The first problem that confronted us was the years of misconceptions and false realities that surround the Christian world and choke faith; Statements like, "You never know what God will do," and "Some people he chooses to heal and some he doesn't." What if my daughter was someone he did not choose to heal?

Some people say that God ordains certain people to travel hard paths for his own greater purposes. Equally frightening were the thoughts in my mind. What if we didn't have enough faith to receive a healing? Did I believe enough? Would Gabrielle? Funny how worrying about my faith levels only made me feel trapped in doubt and unbelief.

It seems that teaching about what Jesus, the Word of John 1:1, says about healing brings some people under condemnation. I've been told that "I prayed and prayed and I didn't get healed. Are you saying there is something wrong with me because I wasn't healed?" Or maybe people just think you are being self-righteous and condescending. I cannot answer for other people or their situations. That is a personal place between them and God. I can only determine to press in my walk with him.

How did all these conflicting teachings start? How did we go from the vibrant, powerful New Testament church to the confused, divided body we are now? The early church was filled with the Spirit and followed Jesus's straightforward command in Matthew 10:7–8,

> **And as ye go, preach, saying the Kingdom of heaven is at hand. Heal the sick, cleanse the lepers, raise the dead, cast out devils: freely ye have received, freely give.**

And in the great commission of Mark 16:15–18,

> **And he said unto them, Go ye into all the world and preach the gospel to every creature. He that believeth and is baptized shall be saved; but he that believeth not shall be damned. And these signs shall follow them that believe; In my name shall they cast out devils; they shall speak with new tongues; they shall take up serpents; and if they drink any deadly thing, it shall not hurt them; they shall lay hands on the sick and they shall recover.**

The early church knew what they were sent to do and they did it. But as the years went by most of the apostles and evangelists and lay people who knew their God were gone. Jesus even warned the great church of Ephesus to return to their first love or he would remove their candlestick out of its place (Rev. 2:1-7).

They were doing many commendable things. They were laboring for him. He did not say they weren't saved and going to heaven. They had lost that first love of just wanting to be with Jesus, to talk with him, to think, and share about him every moment of their lives.

He was telling them that without that type of walk with Jesus, their church would not remain the strongest church of the first century and be the living presence of Jesus to the pagan world. They would not be doing the works of Jesus as they were commanded to do. Gradually the fire of the early church dimmed. That church in Ephesus is no more.

The historian Eusebius reported that about the year 312 Constantine, the current Caesar, believed he saw Christ in the sky. Instead of persecuting the Christians as they had for 300 years, he eventually decreed that everyone had to be a Christian. Now during the first 300 years, Christians would rather burn or be fed to lions than to denounce their faith and follow another god. Persecution kept them on their knees and relying on the one true God. But pagans had no such reservations about changing "religions" if it meant saving their lives or giving them favor with people. So, pagans joined an organization without ever having given their hearts and lives to a living Christ and Messiah. With them came many of the pagan ceremonies and traditions that now are part of the church.

In American history, the Puritans did the same thing to the church. They came to the new world with such high principles and goals. As the years went by, they demanded that no one could hold public office or have a prominent position unless they were part of the church. So people signed on the dotted line without ever having had a personal encounter with Jesus Christ. Eventually all you had to do to qualify was be born into a family that professed Christ. So, leaders began heading the church who were themselves unsaved. They knew little or nothing about healing.

When the sick were brought to this kind of church for prayer and laying on of hands, the leaders dutifully performed their rituals, but people were generally not healed. How could this be explained? A new doctrine had to be devised that said, "Well, it must not have been God's will to heal that person," and then, "It is not God's will to heal everyone." They totally ignored the fact that nowhere in the Bible did Jesus ever expound that belief. In fact, the only place where he could do no mighty miracle was in Nazareth because of their own unbelief. (Mark 6:5–6) Rather than examine the word and their own understanding of the word, people are condemned as being fanatics who would dare question the sovereignty of God.

They quote, "The secret things belong to the Lord our God", but forget the remainder of the verse that says, "but those things, which are revealed, belong unto us and to our children for ever that we may do all the words of this law" (Deut. 29:29).

Jesus taught, "I will utter things which have been kept secret from the foundations of the world" (Matt. 13:35).

Paul quoted from Isaiah 64:4 when he wrote II Corinthians 2:9–12,

> **But as it is written, Eye has not seen, nor ear heard, neither have entered into the heart of man, the things which God has prepared for them that love him.** *But God has revealed them to us by his Spirit:* **[italic is my emphasis] for the Spirit searcheth all things, yea, and the deep things of God. For what man knows the things of a man, except the spirit of man which is in him? Even so the things of God knoweth no man, but the Spirit of God. Now we have received, not the spirit of the world, but the spirit which is of God, that we might know the things that are freely given to us of God.**

It became more comforting to the church to shift responsibility for healing on to God. If it is his will, someone gets healed. If not, God has his reasons unknown to us. It became totally God's responsibility to heal and apparently he did not care to do it very often. Some people truly feel they believed and got the answer no. Some people believe that the age of miracles ended with the apostles.

I remembered as a young person, I grabbled with these same questions and how they fit with what the word of God says. I once asked a pastor about the verse in John 15:7. It seemed so straightforward.

> **If ye abide [dwell continually] in me, my words abide [dwell continually] in you, ye shall ask what ye will and it will be done unto you.**

I asked the minister, if this verse was true, why did we see so few miracles or healings today? It would seem, I said, that the answer had to be in the abiding. He laughed and patted me on the shoulder and gave me no answer. Even as a teenager, I knew that was because he didn't have one.

Have we become so proud of our Christianity that there is not room to learn and grow? God forbid. Lester Sumrall, the great man of God who wrote *Pioneers of Faith*, said,

> **The majority of people throughout Church history never move beyond their first blessing from God-the salvation experience….Once the average believer get in a groove, that is exactly where he or she dies. We are creatures of habit. We move ahead in almost everything except God. People, especially leadership, are embarrassed to admit they don't know everything about God and His Word." (Sumrall, p. 189)**

He goes on to say, "In the beginning of every revival, the poor and the humble are the ones to receive first. They are the people ready and eager to learn at Jesus's feet."

The truth is that there are things of God that we do not understand in this life and sometimes Satan does temporarily win. He comes to steal, kill, and destroy (John 10:10). My family needed to understand and be convinced about the things of God that are given to us. I pictured the woman with the issue of blood (Matt. 9:20-22), who against the laws of her day, pushed through the crowds to reach Jesus. Nothing would deter her until she received her healing. Or the Syrophenician woman (Matt. 15:22–28) with a demonic child who seemingly took verbal abuse, prejudice, and was even compared to a dog, but refused to leave without her healing for her child. I was one of those women. Why not? Why not push through and be determined to touch Jesus? The answers could not come from great sermons, vain traditions, or even other people's testimonies or opinions. The answers all start and finish in The Word of God, Jesus.

Chapter Two
In the Beginning

The entire Bible is the story of the creation and redemption of mankind. In Genesis we see that God created man in the image and likeness of God, and that the Father, the Son, and the Holy Spirit agreed that it was good.

> **Let us make man in our image after our likeness: and let them have dominion over the fish of the sea and over the fowl of the air, and over the cattle, and over all the earth, and over every creeping thing that creepeth upon the earth. Genesis 1:26**

That was God's plan from the beginning, but man was not content to live in paradise. God allowed his children to have free will and with that free will they chose to listen to Satan.

I John 2:15–17 speaks of their condition then and now.

> **Love not the world, neither the things that are in the world. If any man love the world, the love of the Father is not in him. For all that is in the world, the lust of the flesh, and the lust of the eyes, and the pride of life, is not of the Father, but is of the world. And the world passeth away,**

and the lust thereof; but he that doeth the will of God abideth forever.

Eve saw the forbidden fruit in the garden. Her flesh wanted to taste it. It was pleasant to her eyes and she wanted to gain the wisdom which the serpent said would be hers. She took it and gave it to her husband and they both ate it (Gen. 3:6).

So, sin came into the world and with it disease, death, and destruction. But from the beginning of time, God had a plan of redemption and restoration. It is found in Genesis to Revelations. The blood, which had to be shed first in lambs and goats, was later shed with the blood of his own son, Jesus.

Before the fall of mankind, man had the ability to walk and talk with God. There was no separation from God, no sickness, no physical death, no shame. In fact, man had even no knowledge of evil. Satan was not the prince of this world. Adam was. He had dominion over everything on the earth. Adam lost everything in his fall and gained spiritual death, sickness, and physical death. This was never God's plan for mankind, his creation made to be like Him.

Still, in the fallen state, God made covenants with his people, including Adam, Noah, Abraham, Moses. This is "a scarlet thread" from Genesis to Revelations revealing the blood covenants. He gave them promises on the condition that they obey the word. When Moses led the children of Israel out of Egypt, God said in Exodus 15:26,

> **If thou wilt diligently hearken to the voice of the Lord thy God, and will do that which is right in his sight, and wilt give ear to his commandments, and keep all his statutes, I will put** *none of these diseases* **on thee, which I have brought upon the Egyptians** *for I am the Lord that healeth thee.* **[Italic is my emphasis]**

Deuteronomy 28 listed the blessings and curses that God stated would come in this fallen world. Verses 1–14 lists all the blessings and verses 15–68 the curses. Several of the curses involved physical and mental sickness.

- Pestilence: (v. 21) the plague
- Consumption: (v. 22) a progressive wasting away of the body especially from pulmonary tuberculosis
- Inflammation and extreme burning (v. 22)
- Blastings: (v. 22) the blight or cankerous disease, infestation
- Mildews: (v. 22) paleness or yellowish from drought
- Blotch of Egypt: (v. 27) boils like in Egypt
- Emerods: (v. 27) tumors
- The Scab: (v.27) scurvy
- The Itch: (v. 27) scratching from an itch that cannot be healed
- Madness: (v. 28) mental illness
- Blindness: (v. 28)
- Astonishment of the heart: (v. 28) bewilderment, despair
- Every sickness and every plague not written in the book (v. 60,61)

These curses are due to the fall of man and by mankind continuing not to "hearken unto the voice of the Lord thy God, to observe and do all his commandments and his statutes which I command you this day..." (Deut. 28: 1, 15).

Deuteronomy 29:9 says,

Keep therefore the words of this covenant and do them that you may prosper in all that you do.

We understand that this old world is fallen and cursed by sin and depravity. It was never God's plan or intention to bring sickness to mankind. Man was made in his image. He did make a way of escape for the Old Testament followers of him. Sickness and disease are the consequential result in this world of mankind's depravation and disobedience.

Now listen to the good news of the New Testament:

Christ has redeemed us from the curse of the law. Galatians 3:13

According to Merriam-Webster Dictionary to redeem something is to buy it back, free it from what distresses or harms, free from captivity by payment of ransom, to extricate from or help overcome something detrimental, to release from blame, to free from the consequences of sin.

Blotting out the handwriting of ordinances that was against us, which was contrary [an enemy] to us, and took it out of the way, nailing it to his cross; And having spoiled principalities and powers, he made a show of them openly, triumphing over them in it. Colossians 2:14-15

Praise God! That understanding alone should start us jumping and praising God for his love and goodness toward us. We have been freed from the curses of the law! That includes all the sickness and disease listed in Deuteronomy 28.

Romans 5:12 says,

Wherefore, as by one man, sin entered the world, and death by sin; and so death passed to all men for all have sinned.

Romans 5:17 and 19 continues,

For if by one man's offense death reigned by one; much more they which receive abundance of grace and of the gift of righteousness shall reign in life by one, Jesus Christ…For as by one man's disobedience many were made sinners, so by the obedience of one shall many be made righteous.

Romans 6:14 repeats, "For ye are not under the law, but under grace."

During Jesus's ministry on earth, he went teaching and preaching and healing *all* that were oppressed of the devil [Matt. 4:23, Matt. 9:35, Acts 10:38]. Some of the arguments that people make today are, "Well, we aren't Jesus" and that he was only talking about being free from our sins, not sickness.

He commanded us to go do the things we saw him do and greater than these would we do, because we do them in his name (John 14:12). Many people thank him for salvation, but do not believe healing is still part of the covenant promised to us. Can it be that we just cannot believe him? Is it too good to be true?

Listen to Matthew 8:16–17,

When the even was come, they brought unto him many that were possessed with devils; and he cast out the spirits with his word, *and healed all that were sick***: That it might be fulfilled which was spoken by Esaias the prophet, saying, Himself took our infirmities and bare our sicknesses. [Italic is my emphasis]**

This scripture refers both to physical and mental healing and confirms that was the promise given Isaiah (Isa. 53:5). That is what infirmities [weaknesses, diseases, sicknesses] and sicknesses [diseases] mean. I do not understand why Christians feel the need to discredit what the word says and believe for less than what is theirs. Why argue against the goodness and mercy of God? Why not believe The Word, Jesus (John 1:1)?

> **For I came down from heaven, not to do mine own will, but the will of him that sent me.**
>
> **John 6:38**

I once heard someone say to me, "Jesus said it. I believe it. That settles it." Simple maybe, but then even children could understand and receive from Jesus. Perhaps that is why he told us to become as little children and enter into his kingdom (Matt. 18:3).

Hebrews 8:6 says, "But now has he [Jesus] obtained a more excellent ministry, by how much also he is the mediator of a better covenant, which was established upon better promises." In the old covenant, God said he would put none of these diseases on them. And this is the better covenant!

And remember the promise of God in Psalms 89:34,

> **My covenant will I not break, nor alter the thing that is gone out of my lips.**

And Psalms 105:8,

> **He hath remembered his covenant forever, the word which he commanded to a thousand generations.**

He made a covenant with us signed in the blood of his own son. We must decide whether we can believe it and receive it. Remember these important words from Numbers 23:19,

> **God is not a man that he should lie; neither the son of man that he should repent: Hath he said,**

and shall he not do it? Or hath he spoken, and shall he not make it good?

And what was this blood covenant of better promises that Jesus made with us? He went to the cross as a sacrificial, spotless lamb.

We being dead to sins, should live unto righteousness: by whose stripes ye were healed.
I Peter 2:24

We who are born again accepted God's word by faith alone that we are cleansed from our sins. We live in renewed fellowship with God and have a future in heaven. We do not see anything that immediately convinces us that this is true. Faith that is seen is not faith.

We walk by faith, and not by sight.
II Corinthians 5:7

The Spirit brings light for us to know these invisible things. Later we see manifestations of a changed life and a heart toward God.

The same is true of healing. We have to accept the promise by faith, without seeing physical manifestations. We believe it, because God said it, and he cannot lie. We believe it because we believe The Word, Jesus.

I love what Smith Wigglesworth, the great minister of faith, said, "I am not moved by my emotions, what I feel, what I think, or what I see. I am moved by the Word of God." That man saw many, great miracles of God in his lifetime.

Jesus said he only did what he saw the Father do (John 5:19). He then went on to say in John 14:12–13,

Verily, verily, I say unto you, He that believeth on me, the works that I do shall he do also; and

greater works than these shall he do, because I go to my Father. And whatsoever ye shall ask in my name, that will I do, that the Father may be glorified in the Son.

Unless you become fully convinced that it is God's perfect will for you to be healed, you will never be able to stand in faith and fight the good fight of faith. God is not a respecter of persons. His name is "I AM", not I was. If he could keep the children of Israel without a sickly one among them (Ps. 105:37), how much more is available to people of the new and better covenant?

Don't have faith in your own level of faith. You don't try to psych yourself up to believe. Your faith is in a person. Your faith is in the very character and nature and power of the Almighty God who cannot lie. Your faith is in the promises of his word. His word can be believed more than the doctors or even your dearest loved ones.

Let God be true, but every man a liar. Rom. 3:4

Remember, this is not hand-to-hand combat with Satan. You will need to take your position, seated in the heavenlies with Christ Jesus. You will need to pray and understand the words of Ephesians 1:18–22,

The eyes of your understanding being enlightened; that ye may know what is the hope of his calling, and what the riches of the glory of his inheritance in the saints, and what is the exceeding greatness to us-ward who believe, according to the working of his mighty power, which he wrought in Christ, when he raised him from the dead, and set him at his own right hand in the heavenly places, *Far Above* all principality and power, and might, and dominion, and *every name* that is named, not only in this world, but the world to come. And hath put *all things under*

his feet, and gave him to be the head over all things to the church. [**Italic is my emphasis**]

Gabrielle and I read that F.F. Bosworth, who wrote the great book, *Christ the Healer,* said, "If you must doubt something, doubt your doubts, because they are unreliable, but never doubt God or His Word." (p.14)

We spoke that phrase to ourselves many times in the days that followed, until it took root and bore precious fruit.

Chapter Three
The Healings by Jesus

In my study of the word, I found that there are about 19 individual healings of Jesus mentioned in the New Testament, plus several casting out of the demons, which were causing the illness or mental disorder, plus incidents of the raising of the dead. John told us in his gospel that there were many more.

> **And there are also many other things which Jesus did, which if they should be written every one, I suppose that even the world itself could not contain the books that should be written. John 21:25**

Since the writers of the gospel only chose these examples, I believe they must be worth studying as examples of healing to us. What I say has little bearing on anything. It is only what God said through his word that can change situations and hearts. It is my sincere prayer that you will study these portions of scripture for yourself.

> **Faith cometh by hearing, and hearing the word of God. Romans 10:17**

Meditate on each of these examples given to us. See yourself being there with Jesus and hear his words. Let us hear the word of God with open hearts and minds.

1. Healing the Nobleman's Son John 4:4–54

Jesus had just started his ministry when he was approached by a nobleman who had traveled a distance, searching for Jesus to heal his sick son who was about to die. He asked Jesus to come with him back to his house to heal the child. Jesus said,

Except you see signs and wonders, you will not believe.

The Nobleman did not understand what Jesus meant and pleaded again for his son's life. Jesus answered with

Go thy way. Your child lives.

Now this is where most of us miss it. We would keep on begging and pleading to get Jesus to come with us. Jesus wanted the man to know that if he said it, it was done. Jesus does not want us to always look for signs and wonders before we can believe. We do not always have to stand in a prayer line and receive some physical affirmation. He wants us to get to the place where we believe and stand on his word alone.

To the man's credit he believed what Jesus said and left. As simple as that. He just believed and went home. As he was approaching home, his servants told him that the son lived. He asked them when it happened and they said, "Yesterday at the seventh hour," just the same time Jesus that said the word, "Your child lives."

Jesus understands that we want something physical to happen before we can believe. The nobleman wanted a sign of Jesus's presence in his home. Jesus knew that all that was needed was his word.

He sent his word, and healed them, and delivered them from their destructions. Psalms 107:20

2. The demonic healed Mark 1:23–28 and Luke 4:33–37

While in a synagogue in Capernaum, Jesus encountered a man possessed with a "spirit of an unclean devil." The demonic spirit recognized Jesus and began to shout in a loud voice that he knew that Jesus was the Holy One of God. Jesus only said,

Hold your peace and come out of him.

Jesus knew his authority was given to him by God. He knew he was given power and dominion over every foul demonic spirit. He commanded the spirit to stop talking. He refused to listen to the foolish, empty words of the devil. And we should not either.

As a psychiatric home care nurse, I have seen people tormented by foul devils. I remember going into one home where the man was pacing and holding his head. He told me that "voices" were telling him to take a knife and kill himself. He even pointed to the place where the demon was standing, mocking him. I turned to that place, even though I saw nothing, and commanded that demon to shut up and leave my patient's home immediately. The patient relaxed and said it was gone. We have been given the command from Jesus to cast out demons and the necessary power and authority to do it. We have nothing to be afraid of from Satan, unless of course, we don't know who we are in Christ.

3. Peter's Mother-in-law Matthew 8:14–15, Mark 1:29–31, Luke 4:38–39

Capernaum was Jesus's headquarters. After preaching to a great multitude, he went into Peter's home for rest. When he got there, Peter's mother-in-law was lying in bed sick with a fever. The word says Jesus took her hand and lifted her up. He rebuked the fever and it immediately left her. She was able to get up and minister to Jesus and the disciples.

It strikes me is that this older woman was lying in bed and she could have wanted to be allowed to stay there. Certainly we have all been there. Sometimes it takes less effort to lie there and be sick than to believe for healing.

Working in a Christian school, students would come to me, saying they were sick and wanting to go home. When I told them that I would pray for them, they would often turn away disgusted, say, "Never mind," and return to their class. Why? Because sometimes we want to be sick. We may not even realize it. Sometimes we want self-pity or attention. Sometimes we want to get out of bothersome life situations, like school or work. Sometimes in our weakened condition we just want to be left alone.

Praise God that Peter's mother-in-law was not one of those kinds of people and Jesus did not look at her with pity or indulgence. He rebuked the disease. She received the healing and gave God the glory by continuing to serve him.

4. The Leper Healed Matthew 8:2–4, Mark 1:40–42, Luke 5:12–14

This is the story of Jesus being approached by a man, as Luke the physician described, being "full of leprosy." Leprosy had to have been one of the most terrifying diseases in its time. It disfigured the body and filled the person with pain, both physical and emotional. People feared catching the disease to the extent that sufferers were shunned and banished from society. Yet this man risked approaching Jesus and humbled himself by falling on his face before him.

His words to Jesus are so important. "Lord, *if you will*, you can make me clean." [Italic is my emphasis] Notice first he recognized the Lordship of Jesus and Jesus's ability to heal and cleanse. What he wasn't sure of, what so many today are unsure of, is the question would Jesus choose to heal them? Most believers and many unbelievers agree that miracles still exist today and that Jesus has the power to heal. What they fear to ask is *will* Jesus heal me?

Jesus did the unthinkable to a person with leprosy. He reached out and touched the man. The gospel writer Mark added the phrase, "moved with compassion." I can imagine what that must have felt like to a man who was shunned and untouched by others. It must have been so long since he felt love and compassion from anyone. Jesus simply answered, "I will. Be clean."

Understand what the apostle Peter learned in Acts 10:34,

Of a truth I perceive that God is no respecter of persons.

The all-important question is not *can* God heal, but *will he*? Until you can hear in your spirit and not doubt his words, "I will. Be healed", you will not be able to receive in faith what is given you. You must forever settle in your mind that it is God's will to heal you and Satan's will that you not be healed. How do you get it settled in your mind? Renew your mind with the Word of God. Say what he says. Believe you receive because he said it.

Therefore I say unto you, whatsoever things ye desire, when ye pray, believe that ye receive them and ye shall have them. Mark 11:24

5. The Paralytic Man Healed Matthew 9:2–8, Mark 2:2–12, Luke 5:18–26

This is an important story of the miraculous power of God. Most Christians know the story of the paralyzed man whose friends carried him to Jesus. They had to lower him through the roof to get to Jesus because of the great crowd surrounding him. Jesus looked at the man, saw the friends' faith, and told him his sins were forgiven. Apparently Jesus knew that the sin problem was the greatest issue in that man's life.

As usual, the "religious" people were outraged. Who did Jesus think he was to forgive someone's sins? Jesus knew their thoughts and openly addressed them with a question. What was easier to do, heal someone's disease or forgive his or her sins?

> **But that ye may know that the Son of man hath power on earth to forgive sins, (he saith to the sick of the palsy,) I say unto thee, Arise, and take up thy bed, and go thy way unto thine house.**
>
> **Mark 2:10, 11**

Do you see the significance here? Salvation is a miracle. Healing is a miracle. Both are provided by Jesus. Both have to be received by our faith. Neither are too hard for God. Both give God glory.

T.L. Osborn made a great point in his wonderful book, *Healing the Sick.*

> **How many would be saved if they never heard a message on salvation? Or if, when the message of salvation was addressed, the points expounded were (1) Maybe it isn't God's will to save you. (2) Perhaps your sin is for God's glory. (3) Perhaps God is using your sin to chastise you. (4) Be patient in your sin until God wills to save you. (5) The days of miracle conversion is past. [Page 28]**

We need to accept that it is God's will for you to receive the salvation he provided through Jesus Christ. Providing healing is no harder for him than forgiving your sins. That paralyzed man was immediately healed and God received the glory from the healed and forgiven man.

6. Man at the Pool of Bethesda John 5:2–15

In Jerusalem there was a pool where sick people waited for the stirring of the water because they believed that an angel occasionally stirred it. When that happened, whoever was the first into the pool received their healing. One man was sick thirty-eight years and now was unable to walk. Jesus saw him lying there and knew that he had been waiting there a long time for his miracle. Notice the question that Jesus asked that man.

Wilt thou be made whole?

Jesus still asks us that same question. I was at a home of a dear Christian couple. The husband had been sick most of his life and was now bedridden. The wife asked me to pray with him and she asked him what he would like us to pray. He said, "I'd like to be a little better." The wife later expressed her frustration to me by explaining that all his life all he ever wanted was to be "a little" better. He never could believe for "wholeness", because he felt his sickness was the consequence of his younger worldly life. He even feared that he might be tempted to return to that former life, if he received a full healing.

"Will you be made whole?" seems like a strange question to ask a man who was sick for thirty-eight years and spent his time waiting for pool water to stir. Jesus wanted the man to be honest with himself and identify his problem and the solution. The man was able to tell Jesus that he really wanted to be healed, but could not get into the pool in time.

Jesus saw the diseased man's heart and told him to pick up his bed and walk. The man could have reminded Jesus that he could not walk or he could have been afraid to try, but he believed Jesus's words and moved in faith. That man immediately received his healing.

When the religious leaders saw the man was healed, their main concern was that he was carrying his bed on the Sabbath. He explained that he was just doing what the man, who healed him, told him to do. He did not even know who Jesus was. Jesus found this man later and told him in verse 14,

Behold, thou art made whole: Sin no more, lest a worse thing come unto thee.

This is a controversial statement in today's church. There is such a thing as sin. Jesus healed him, but knew that the man needed to make spiritual corrections in his life to stay well. It did not mean that Jesus would punish him, but that the devil would be able to attack him again. He could remove himself from the covenant covering. We need to judge ourselves and realize that sin affects our health.

So many times in my life I have seen a miraculous healing given to a person with limited understanding of God's word, simply because of the goodness and mercy of God. When that person receives their healing and does not correct their life by learning about their healer, Jesus, they open themselves up to be attacked again. This time they may have no faith or strength to resist the devil.

We need to want our healing so that we can complete our God-given assignment on earth. That man at the pool now was able to tell others that he met Jesus and knew who his healer was. Jesus wants to heal us so that we can give glory to God and serve Him.

7. Healing the Withered Hand Matthew 12:9–13, Mark 3:1–5, Luke 6:6–10

Jesus entered a synagogue on the Sabbath. The religious leaders asked him (trying to trick him into doing wrong), if it was lawful to heal someone on the Sabbath. Jesus has a brilliant mind and according to Matthew, turned the situation around by asking them a question.

What man shall there be among you, that shall have one sheep, and if it falls into a pit on the Sabbath day, will he not lay hold on it, and lift it out? How much then is a man better than a sheep?

Luke added to that question,

> **Is it lawful to do good on the Sabbath days, or to do evil? To save life, or to destroy it?**

The people never answered his question so he answered it himself by example. He told the man with a withered hand to stretch out his hand. Again, the man had to move in faith and obey. Jesus was angry at the accusers because of their "hardness of heart." This man's heart was soft and pliable and he chose to believe Jesus instead of his peers and the religious leaders in his synagogue. He had to stand against the religious distorted rules of keeping the Sabbath. He stretched forth his withered hand. He was healed.

Notice that Jesus said that "doing good" and "saving life" were lawful and right. He said the opposite was true of "doing evil" and "destroying life". Healing is a good thing. Saving someone's life is a good thing. Disease and affliction are evil. They kill and destroy lives. Jesus was all about doing good.

Peter preached,

> **How God anointed Jesus of Nazareth with the Holy Ghost and with power: who went about doing good, and healing all that were oppressed of the devil; for God was with him. Acts 10:38**

The Hebrews writer in Hebrews 13:8 said,

> **Jesus Christ the same yesterday, and to day, and for ever.**

And James added

> **Every good gift and every perfect gift is from above, and cometh down from the Father of lights**

with whom there is no variableness [fickleness], neither shadow of turning [movement even to smallest degree]. James 1:17

Jesus has not changed. He still wants to be good to you. He wants you healed!

8. The Roman Centurion's Servant Matthew 8:5–13, Luke 7:2–10

Israel in the time of Jesus was a nation conquered by the Roman Empire. A Roman Centurion was the symbol of the tyranny of the hated enemy. Centurions were officers and commanded hundreds of men. Luke tells us that this certain centurion had a servant that was "dear" to him, who was sick and ready to die. He had heard about Jesus and sent for Jewish elders and asked about Jesus. These elders told Jesus that the centurion was a good man who was just and honorable to the Jewish nation.

Jesus started out with the elders toward the centurion's home when he was intercepted by a message from the centurion saying,

> **Lord, trouble not thyself: for I am not worthy that thou shouldest enter under my roof: Therefore neither thought I myself worthy to come unto thee: but say in a word, and my servant shall be healed. For I also am a man set under authority, having under me soldiers, and I say to one, Go and he goeth; and to another, Come and he cometh; and to my servant, Do this and he doeth it.**
>
> **Luke 7:6–8**

Read those words over several times until the importance really sinks in. Jesus turned to the crowd and said he had never found such *great faith* in all of Israel. That servant received his healing immediately due to the uncompromising faith of someone who loved him.

> **And Jesus unto the centurion, Go your way; and as thou hast believed, so be it done unto you. Matt. 8:13**

If that statement was made today by anyone other than Jesus, people would be offended. They would think Jesus must be one of the "faith people", who emphasizes your faith part in the healing process. Nevertheless, he made it clear. The man believed in Jesus's desire and power to heal. He believed Jesus had only to speak the word and it was done. He did not need a sign or a wonder. He understood the principle of delegated authority because he lived it. Then he made the all-important step of putting corresponding action to his faith. He went home in peace knowing his servant was healed.

> **But wilt thou know, o vain man, that faith without works is dead? James 2:20**

Since I was a little girl, when someone got seriously ill, I always heard, "Remember Brother So-and-so. He was one of the Godliest men I knew and he died. He even went to an Oral Roberts meeting for healing and was prayed for, but he died." The implication was that it was God's will and timing for him to die and God doesn't heal everyone for reasons unknown to us. It wasn't until years later that my father talked to me about the incident. He told me that the good brother went to the healing service only to please his friends and family, but he told my dad that he knew he wasn't going to get healed. He didn't get healed. He died leaving a wife and young son and a legacy of confusion to others about healing. He died believing in his salvation and heaven, but not his healing. He got what he was believing. Think about that!

Personally, my family was convinced by the word to believe it was God's perfect will to heal Gabrielle. When asked by people about her condition, we said, "The doctors say she has lymphoma, but Jesus says she's healed." It wasn't empty words. It was putting action to our faith. We believed totally in Jesus's word and we received what we believed.

9. The Blind and Mute Demoniac Matthew 12:22, Luke 11:14–16

Then was brought unto him one possessed with a devil, blind, and dumb: and he healed him, insomuch that the blind and dumb both spake and saw. Matthew 12:22

In this case, Jesus recognized the fact that illness was due to demonic spirits working in the man. That he healed him is not unusual, but the responses that occurred afterward were. It says "all the people" were amazed and said, "Is this not the son of David?" The simple folk were able to see the healing and recognize Jesus as the promised Messiah. Meanwhile the Pharisees, the religious class of people who dedicated themselves to following the law, missed it entirely. Instead of rejoicing in the freeing of this tormented man, they decided that because the healing did not occur in the manner and traditions they were used to, it had to be of the devil.

Beware of the Pharisees of our day. They may even be sincere in their beliefs, but they attack anything out of their realm of understanding. They may smile and say, "Stay away from those fanatics," or "Miracles have been done away with after the apostles." Their lack of understanding of God and their pride which forbids them from learning more, hurt a lot of wonderful people who start out in faith and then are discouraged.

(There is a similar story of another mute man possessed of a devil in Matthew 9:32–34. This is not to imply that all muteness is causes by demonic possession. In this case it is clear that there was a demon causing the impairment. To be healed, the man had to be free of the causal spirit.)

It appears obvious by the word that many sicknesses are due to demonic spirits. Certainly, Satan is behind all sickness and disease, since God is incapable of creating evil.

One of my beloved aunts was diagnosed with breast cancer. We went to a ladies breakfast and sat next to the woman speaker. She shared with us her belief that there was a tenacious, demonic spirit with cancer that worked to wear down a person until they were too tired to fight. Together in the name of Jesus we rebuked that demonic spirit working to give my aunt breast cancer. My aunt chose to believe God and not to undergo surgery or treatments. She just went on with her life and was healed of the cancer.

10. The Gadarenes Demoniacs At The Tomb Matthew 8:28–34, Mark 5-1–20, Luke 8:26–39

Matthew cites two men, while Mark and Luke speak about only one man. In all cases the description is the same. The man was totally possessed by devils. He was a wild man, naked and living in tombs, who could not even be restrained with chains. Matthew says the man was so fierce that people were unable to pass near him.

Even the demons recognized who Jesus was and called him "Son of God." They also knew that their time for judgment and torment was coming. Just recognizing the Christ did not make them followers of Jesus, any more than it does us.

They knew that they were powerless against the authority of Jesus to cast them out of the man they possessed. Therefore, they asked to be sent into a herd of swine. Jesus said one word, "Go," and the demons left the man, entered the swine, and their insane spirits sent the swine right off the edge of the cliff.

Average people become frightened by the thought of demons and their ability to possess someone. Hollywood makes horror movies about it so it will appear to be fantasy. Two great errors in thought are that demons do not exist, while the other is to overemphasize them. Jesus knows the demonic spirits are real and present in our world today. Most of the severely mentally ill people with whom I worked also knew it. Demonic spirits continue to torment and rob people of the life God intended for them. Jesus modeled our response: don't be afraid, know your authority in Jesus, and cast them out.

11. The Woman Afflicted With An Issue of Blood Matthew 9:20–22, Mark 5:25–34, Luke 8:43-–48

Jesus was on his way to heal a little girl. The crowds crushed around him wanting to see him perform miracles. In that crowd was a woman who had been bleeding for twelve years. According to Jewish law she was considered unclean and was not allowed to touch other people. The scripture tells us that she had suffered many things by the procedures of physicians, spent all her money on treatments, yet only got worse. This is a familiar situation even in modern medical science today.

> **For** *she said within herself* **(Italic is my emphasis),**
> **if I may but touch his garment, I shall be whole.**
> **Matthew 9:21**

She touched the hem of his garment. Although many people thronged around him, he felt that one touch of faith in the middle of a pressing, spectator crowd. He felt healing flow out of him. He asked who had touched him and looked around to see the woman who confessed her whole story to him. Listen to his words.

> **Daughter, thy faith hath made thee whole; Go**
> **in peace, and be whole of thy plague. Mark 5:34**

In the Old Testament Malachi prophesied in chapter 4:2a,

But unto you that fear [reverence] my name shall the Sun of righteousness arise with healing in his wings [the border of a garment].

Had she known that ancient prophesy about healing or had she just listened to Jesus's words and believed in him? She believed enough to stake her reputation and life on him. She believed and Jesus said it was her faith that made her well. Jesus is still looking for that type of bold faith that will press through the throng of unbelievers, sign seekers, or pious people of tradition and laws, and choose to believe. Believe against the prevalent thinking of the day. Believe that your God is able and willing to heal. He said that it was *her faith* that healed her. This can be a controversial statement to a church that does not want to accept their responsibility to have faith in God.

I also want to point out his statement "Go in peace and be whole of your plague." She now had to receive that healing and believe for wholeness. This is where many good Christians miss it.

I nursed a lovely widow woman who had a terminal diagnosis of gastric cancer and was on chemotherapy and radiation. One night in prayer I felt the Lord speak to me to tell her that she was healed. I questioned it at first because she was 80 years old and ready to meet the Lord, but I obeyed and told her. She immediately said she believed it and we had a time of rejoicing. When her next appointment came, she received the news that her scan showed no signs of cancer! However the doctors wanted to keep her on the chemotherapy "prophylactically", just in case the cancer returned. Under pressure from her family and against her own judgment, she agreed to continued medical treatment. The cancer never came back, but one day while visiting her, she didn't know who I was. She had to be admitted to a nursing home with "chemo-brain" damage. She eventually died there. I praise God that she is in heaven, but I know she did not have to end her days lonely and confused.

12. Daughter of Jairus Matthew 9:18–19, 23–26, Mark 5:22–24, 35–43, Luke 8:41–42, 49–56

This was an interrupted miracle; interrupted by the woman mentioned previously. Jesus had been teaching the multitudes when a ruler of a synagogue came worshipping Jesus and told him that his daughter was at the point of dying. He believed that if Jesus could just come and lay hands on her, she would live. Jesus started to follow him, but the woman with the issue of blood touched him. As a parent who knows the feelings of having a sick child, that delay must have been excruciating. When they did get on the path again, a messenger from his home arrived to say the girl had died. Circumstances did not move Jesus, no matter how hopeless they appeared. He immediately said powerful words to the ruler,

Be not afraid, only believe. Mark 5:36

Jesus knew that fear is the enemy of faith. My husband knew that too when he immediately told me we did not have time to get into fear and doubts over our daughter's diagnosis. Jesus also knew that the multitudes would not be able to believe, so he only took Peter, James, and John with him. When you need to believe God for something supernatural, move away from people who cannot share your faith and may offer you words of logic or sympathy contrary to the word of God. This is the time to find like-minded Christians to stand with you who will agree with what God says. When Jesus got to the house and heard the mourning, he did not give the people sympathy. Sympathy sounds kind, but can actually destroy a person trying to believe God.

Give place for the maid is not dead but sleeps.

While the spectators scorned the words of Jesus, he took only the mother and father, Peter, James, and John into the girl's room. He knew that they would not hinder him with their unbelief. He took her by the hand and commanded that she arise. Immediately she responded to the voice of God's authority on earth.

God has given that same authority to us as followers of him.

> **And as ye go, preach, saying The kingdom of heaven is at hand. Heal the sick, cleanse the lepers, raise the dead, cast out devils: freely ye have received, freely give. Matt 10:7, 8**

This was a command, not a request, from Jesus. We have a long way to go to do what he said we should be doing. That is not an excuse, just a sad, but true statement.

13. Two blind men Matthew 9:27–31

Jesus had just left the home of Jairus when two blind men started following him loudly yelling "Son of David, have mercy on us." Son of David was the expression used for the Messiah. These men knew who Jesus was. Apparently, Jesus just ignored them and kept on walking, until he came to the house where he stayed while in Capernaum. These blind men did not give up, but persistently charged after Jesus and followed him into the house.

> **Jesus saith unto them, Believe ye that I am able to do this?**

It seems obvious by their behaviors that they believed that Jesus was the Messiah and that he was able to heal them. Still Jesus asked. He needed their confession of faith to be made with their mouths.

**For with the heart man believeth unto
righteousness; and with the mouth confession is
made unto salvation [deliverance, health, safety].**
Romans 10:10

These men did not have a theological debate about why they
needed to speak the words. They just did it. Then Jesus touched
their eyes and said,

According to your faith be it unto you.

According to *your* faith. They believed in their hearts that they
would receive and confessed it with their mouths. And they received
their sight.

14. The Syrophoenician's Daughter Matthew 15:22–28, Mark 7:25–30

Jesus was traveling along the coast of Tyre and Sidon when a
Canaanite woman, a Gentile, began to cry after him. Her words
were similar to the Jewish blind men.

**Have mercy on me, Oh Lord, thou son of David;
my daughter is grievously vexed [brought under
the power] with a devil.**

What Jesus did here is not consistent with the average Christian's
view of Jesus. However it is totally consistent with who he is. He
told her that he was only sent to the lost sheep of Israel. Jesus is
incapable of lying and certainly would not use a lie to test her faith.
No, it was the truth. Jesus repeatedly told people that he could only
do what the Father told him to do. He was sent as Messiah to the
Jews. Later the disciples that followed him, including us, would be
sent to the Gentiles.

This woman came and worshipped Jesus and continued her petition to the Lord. Still he refused, saying,

It is not meet [appropriate] to take the children's bread and to cast it to the dogs.

Again, Jesus said it and so it was absolutely the truth. He was explaining to her and his disciples that he was sent to the house of Israel and healing was for them. While the term dogs is a harsh word, it is part of the analogy Jesus was making. Still, this woman refused to leave Jesus without her daughter being healed. She demonstrated her faith, sincerity, and humility in her answer.

Yea Lord, yet the dogs eat the crumbs which fall from the master's table.

She did not leave offended. She did not give up. She recognized that she was an unworthy dog under the master's table, but she knew even crumbs from Jesus would heal her daughter.

Jesus answered and said to her, O woman, great is thy faith. Be it unto you even as you will.

Nothing changed with what Jesus had said to her previously. He made it clear that it was her faith that produced the answer she needed. Mark added that Jesus told her to go home because the devil had left her daughter. Without further pleading or asking for assurances, she went home to find her daughter well.

This is the kind of faith Jesus is looking for in each of us. Faith that is sure and unshakeable. Faith that does not take no for an answer!

15. The Deaf Man Mark 7:32–37

Next Jesus went to the Sea of Galilee. There a man, who was deaf and had an impediment in his speech, was brought to him for a healing touch. Jesus took the man away from the crowds, who were there hoping to see something "happen". He put his fingers in the man's ears and spit on the man's tongue. Then he looked to heaven and commanded the ears to open and the tongue to loosen.

This healing is important because it shows us that God is not in a box. If we experienced a healing like that, we might think that we should go around sticking our fingers in every deaf person ears and spitting on their tongues. Jesus was listening to the Father and only did what he heard the Father say. We need to listen to the Holy Spirit in our own lives and follow his direction. Obedience is necessary to see God work in our lives. Do what he tells you to do, even if it seems foolish.

16. The Blind Man at Bethsaida Mark 8:22–26

A similar incident happened in Bethsaida. People brought a blind man to Jesus asking for him to touch him. Again, Jesus led him out of town to a private place. Jesus was not about providing a show for non-believers. He spit on the man's eyes, laid his hands on him, and asked him if he could see. The man said he could see men like trees walking. Jesus again put his hands on the man's eyes and this time the man saw clearly. Again he told the man not to tell anyone. Why? Because Jesus wanted people to follow him as the Messiah, not just for the sign and wonders and gifts.

It is interesting that it would seem that there was not an immediate healing. I have seen bedridden people be healed and still have to build up the muscular strength that had been sapped from them. It would appear that after years of blindness, the man had to give his eyes time to readjust to light.

Rev. Kenneth E. Hagen tells about his healing as a teenager

from the debilitating and terminal illness of congenital heart disease. While he believed that he received his healing, it took time for him to go from bedridden to walking. He kept getting up and moving forward by his faith and not by circumstances or how he felt, until the full strength was manifested. The experience only served to strengthen his faith.

Why did Jesus spit on the man? I don't know and neither do you. He was obedient to his Father. This is our Father's business and we don't have to understand it or try to control it. We have only to obey the directions he gives us.

17. The Epileptic Son Matthew 17:14–21, Mark 9:17–29, Luke 9:37–42

Jesus had just come down from the Mount of Transfiguration with Peter, James, and John. The remaining disciples had been busy trying unsuccessfully to heal a boy. His father described the boy as having a dumb spirit that takes hold of the boy "tearing him." This spirit caused him to foam at the mouth, gnash his teeth, and often even throw himself into a fire or into water. The father had brought his son to the disciples, but they could not cast out the spirit. Jesus spoke to his followers.

> **O faithless and perverse [opposing the purposes of God] generation, how long shall I be with you and suffer [put up with] you? Bring the son here.**

If Jesus sounded frustrated here, it may have been because he knew his time on earth was short and his disciples had to learn the truths about whom they are in Christ and the authority given to them. These disciples had witnessed the power of Jesus and had listened to his teachings every day for over two years. They understood what they were supposed to do, but they did not yet grasp the fullness of their delegated authority.

As the boy saw Jesus approaching, the demonic spirit began to tear at the boy and he fell to the ground foaming at the mouth. Jesus knew this was a frightening sight and immediately told the father,

If thou can believe, all things are possible to him that believeth.

The father cried out through his tears, "Lord I believe; help thou my unbelief." We have all felt that way at times when a situation seem impossible in the natural. We want to believe, but know that we need the supernatural help of the Lord. That is the kind of help Jesus is eager to give.

Jesus rebuked the spirit, which caused the spirit to cry out. Before it came out, it convulsed the boy until the boy lay still, looking dead. I have experienced this in my own life when casting out a demonic spirit. The spirit does not go graciously, but often will "tear" at the person before leaving. The freed person may appear exhausted, sweating, and quiet, but smiling. There can be no mistaking the wondrous work of The Lord.

Afterward the disciples asked Jesus why they had been not able to cast out the spirit. Jesus explained to them about their unbelief.

Because of your unbelief: for verily I say to you, If you have faith as a grain of mustard seed, you shall say to his mountain, remove hence to yonder place and it shall remove and nothing shall be impossible to you. However this kind [of unbelief] goes not out but by prayer and fasting. Matt. 17:20–21

There are unfortunately times in our walk that we have spent too much time immersed in the world and not enough time alone with Jesus. We realize our faith is not able to believe for the impossible and we need to hear from God. Nothing substitutes for relationship with God and learning in his presence.

Jesus explained to us in this passage how we could change doubt and unbelief into faith. Fasting and prayer does not change God or his will. It changes us by denying our fleshly desires for a time in order to be in his presence and seek his face. When we spend that kind of quality time with the Lord, we come out like Moses with a glowing face. We have been with God, heard from God, and are convinced of his will. We now know that no demon is a match for the light of God inside us. We may hear specifics about the demon or the illness as God needs to share with us. We are refreshed and ready to resume the works of God.

18. Blind Bartimaeus Mark 10:46–52, Matthew 20:29–34, Luke 18:35–43

Jesus had been ministering around Jericho. The gospels state there was a great number of blind, deaf, and lame people, who sat by the road side begging. Mark tells us that one of these beggars was named Bartimaeus, son of Timaeus. He must have heard about the teachings and miracles of Jesus and recognized him as the Messiah. When he heard that Jesus of Nazareth was passing by, he began to scream out,

Jesus, son of David, have mercy on me.

Can you picture this part? The crowd was shouting for the man to be quiet so they could hear Jesus. He yelled even louder.

Jesus, son of David, have mercy on me.

Jesus commanded the interfering people to tell Bartimaeus to come forward. Bartimaeus threw down his coat and came immediately to Jesus. What is the significance of the coat? Maybe he got rid of any hindrances that would keep him from going quickly to Jesus. Maybe the coat represented his old life of sickness and begging. Perhaps it symbolized his former covering of his own self-righteousness. Whatever the case, he wanted to be free and unencumbered to run to Jesus.

As in other cases, Jesus asked what would appear to be a pointless question to a blind man yelling for mercy.

What will you that I should do unto you? [In other words, what do you want me to do?]

He could have asked for begging money, but Bartimaeus knew what he wanted and asked to receive his sight. This time Jesus didn't touch his eyes or cast out a demon. He simply told the man,

Go your way; *your faith* **(Italic is my emphasis) has made you whole.**

Immediately the man received his sight and began following Jesus. What a great example Bartimaeus is to us. If only all people looked to Jesus today with that simplicity and fervor of heart. He raced to Jesus believing in him as Messiah and healer. Jesus did not have to tell him to go and sin no more. Bartimaeus became a follower of Christ from that time. He glorified God with his eyes and his life of service.

19. Healing Ten Lepers Luke 17:11–19

Jesus entered a village and ten lepers stood "afar off" yelling, "Jesus, Master, have mercy on us." Jesus simply answered,

Go show yourselves to the priests.

The lepers understood the significance of this. According to the Old Testament law, if lepers believed that they were well, they needed to show themselves to the priest for verification. So they knew Jesus was saying they were healed. Still it took faith in the Jesus, The Word of God, to head toward the priest without seeing any visible changes for themselves. They were healed as they went!

And it came to pass, as they went, they were cleansed. And one of them, when he saw that he was healed, turned back, and with a loud voice glorified God. And fell down on his face at his feet, giving him thanks; and he was a Samaritan.

While nine men rushed off to get approved by the priest and reinstated into society, one postponed that for a greater priority. He returned to give God glory and to praise him for his healing before society actually confirmed it. He came back to worship at the feet of Jesus. He was full of thankfulness and joy for the wonderful and unmerited favor shown him. He, who was a Samaritan and considered a second class citizen by the righteous people, recognized just how much compassion and grace he had been given.

Now listen to Jesus's response to this man's worship.

Were there not ten cleansed? But where are the nine? There were not found that returned to give glory to God, save this stranger...Arise, go your way; thy faith has made thee whole.

It must amaze God that we, who have received so much, are thankful so infrequently. Jesus sent the man back on the task of going to the priest, but told the man that his grateful, loving heart had healed more than just leprosy that day. Jesus said the man's faith had made him whole; whole in his spirit, soul, and body. Jesus desires and deserves our praise. Praising God is the greatest antidote to brokenness known to man!

20. Man Blind From Birth John 9:1–41

John expounds at length about this man who was born blind and left to beg on the temple steps. Everyone going into the temple knew him and he was close enough to listen to people speaking in the synagogue.

The disciples asked Jesus about the cause of the man's infirmity. They had learned from the religious leaders about the curses of Deuteronomy. Jesus immediately made it clear that this blindness was not due to the man's or his parents' sin, nor should we look at all sick people that way. Jesus discerned from his Father that while all sickness entered the world through Adam's sin and fall, God does not punished his children by placing sickness and disease on them. Jesus made it clear that even when medical science does not know the cause of an illness, Jesus came to bring life, healing, and grace.

> **But that the works of God should be made manifest in him, I must work the works of Him that sent me, while it is day; Night comes when no man can work. As long as I am in the world, I am the light of the world.**

Some people will argue that God made the man blind just so Jesus could show his power in healing him. The nurse in me knows that sickness, disability, afflictions happen for many reasons. Congenital blindness may be caused by lack of oxygen at birth, genetic damage, heredity, etc. My God is not evil, but good. He doesn't punish a newborn baby just for his own purposes. Sickness happens in this world. Jesus came to free us from it. Jesus said in John 10:10

> **The thief comes not but to steal, and to kill, and to destroy. I am come that they might have life and that they might have it more abundantly.**

Anyone who has ever been sick knows that it is not abundant life. Many a person's faith has been destroyed by religious tradition that says that the sickness was God's appointment and we should be submissive to that act of God. If that was the case, why even ask God for healing? Why take any medical treatment? Jesus clearly said that he came to destroy the works of Satan. He came to give us abundant life. He came to fulfill the words of Isaiah 61:1–3.

Once while he was in the synagogue in Nazareth, the book of Isaiah was handed to him and he opened it to that passage.

The Spirit of the Lord is upon me, because he hath anointed me to preach the gospel to the poor; he has sent me to heal the brokenhearted, to preach deliverance to the captives and recovering of sight to the blind, to set at liberty them that are bruised, to preach the acceptable year of the Lord. And he closed the book, and gave it again to the minister, and sat down. And the eyes of all them that were in the synagogue were fastened on him. And he began to say unto them, This day is this scripture fulfilled in your ears. Luke 4:18–21

If you want to continue to believe God gave the man blindness, the point still is that Jesus did not want him to stay in that state. He spit on the ground, made clay, and put it on the eyes of the man. Then he told him,

Go, wash in the pool of Siloam, which is by interpretation, Sent.

The man was blind and getting to that pool might have been a hard task. Jesus moved with compassion, but not with sympathy. He demands faith. The man moved in faith and obeyed Jesus. It would seem likely that while sitting on those temple steps, he heard the teaching of Jesus and about the miracles performed. He went to wash where he was "Sent" and come back seeing.

The story does not end there. Everyone recognized the man who had been blind and began questioning him. The religious leaders began to interrogate him. He told his story repeatedly, exactly as it happened, but these leaders told him, "This man is not of God," because Jesus healed the man on the sabbath. Then the leaders decided that the man must have not really been blind at all! They called in witnesses to prove this was a con job. The man's parents testified that he had in fact been born blind, but refused to say what happened to him. They seemed to be more afraid of the religious leaders than happy for his healing. How many religious people still refuse to give God glory for miracles, if they do not fit into their ideas and traditions?

The man was again questioned about Jesus and said, "Whether he is a sinner or not, I know not. One thing I know that whereas I was blind, now I see."

After more religious ramblings of the church leaders, he added, "Why this is a marvelous thing; that you know not from where he came, and yet he opened my eyes. Now we know that God doesn't hear sinners: but if any man be a worshipper of God and does His will, He hears him."

The conversation continued until the leadership excommunicated him from the temple. When Jesus heard about it, he found the man and told him that Jesus is the Son of God. The man worshipped him and became a follower of Christ. Organized religion may not have accepted him or his miracle, but praise God, he was accepted by the Beloved One and he could see!

21. Woman With A Spirit of Infirmity Luke 13:10–17

Luke, the physician, tells of another incident that happened when Jesus was teaching in a synagogue on the Sabbath. Women were not allowed to sit in the front with the men, but Jesus saw a woman in the back who was so bent over that she couldn't even lift herself up. An interesting phrase is used here:

A woman which had a spirit of infirmity eighteen years

During my years of working with and praying for the sick, I have come to recognize this spirit of infirmity. When a person has been ill for long periods of time, they cannot even see themselves as well anymore. They become used to the terrible illness, the degradation, and the pain. They begin to accept that this is just the way life is for them. They have given up believing for anything better and so become bound to their illness as a part of themselves. I have seen many of a saint suffer humbly and quietly and I appreciated that they continue to worship God while in pain.

Still, I thank God that Jesus sees everything from a higher plane than we do. He called the woman to break with the tradition in the synagogue and come forward to him. He knew how the religious leaders felt about breaking tradition and healing someone on the Sabbath and this was a woman! Jesus's concern was for the woman and the suffering she had been through for eighteen years. She had the courage and faith to come forward at his command. His words to her were,

Woman, thou are loosed from thine infirmity. And he laid his hands on her and immediately she was made straight and glorified God.

Jesus came to bind the brokenhearted and loose the captives. When Christians get excited about binding and loosing (Matt 18:18), maybe they should remember the context of forgiveness and compassion that Jesus used with those words. He told us that whatsoever we bind or loose on earth, is bound and loosed in heaven.

Maybe we should be using that power on binding the wounds of the brokenhearted and captive people with which we come in contact, and loosening the mercy and love of Jesus on their lives. We, like Jesus, are commissioned in his name to set people free.

The woman glorified God, but the religious rulers were indignant. Jesus called them hypocrites and reminded them that they would be kinder to one of their animals than to this hurting human.

> **Ought not this woman, being a daughter of Abraham, *whom Satan has bound these eighteen years* (Italic emphasis is mine), be loosed from this bond on the Sabbath day?**

Satan caused this spirit of infirmity. He bound her, not God. She was a daughter of Abraham, a worshipper of the God of Israel. For eighteen years Satan had kept her captive to her illness. Jesus came to set her free.

Jesus is the same today. He still wants to set people free, but first we must recognize the spirit of infirmity is from Satan.

> **Jesus Christ the same yesterday, and today, and forever. Hebrews 13:8**

22. The Man With Dropsy Luke 14:1–4

Jesus was invited to eat at the house of a chief Pharisee on the Sabbath. Luke added that the invitation was given so that they could watch Jesus. They wanted to see something with which they could accuse Jesus. It may have been the reason that they also invited a man with dropsy. Dropsy is another word for edema or swelling of the skin. It usually indicates an underlying problem in the circulation or heart, some type of internal infections, and sometimes even malfunctioning organs. Whatever the disease was, the Pharisees knew Jesus would notice it and be too compassionate to let it pass without wanting to heal.

Jesus, of course, knew what they were thinking and asked the Pharisees if it were lawful to heal on the Sabbath. They had no answer. Pharisees rarely do. So Jesus illustrated the answer by taking the man and healing him.

It is interesting to note that even Pharisees understood Jesus's nature and power to heal. They knew that he would use every opportunity to move in compassion. He came preaching and teaching and healing all. He showed mercy and grace and he told us to go and do likewise (Luke 10:37).

In Conclusion:

These examples of healings were recorded so that when Jesus ascended to his Father, his followers would be able to understand his character, principles, and power, and be able to continue his works. We live in a carnal world, surrounded by carnal people and events. It takes more than just saying we believe for a miracle. We have to understand the foundational teachings of Jesus so we can be able to stand in faith and have a basis for our belief.

Jesus shared the parable of the sower sowing the seed in Mark 4, so we could understand that each of us have the opportunity to hear the word. The soil of your heart is what will make a difference. The word never takes hold when the heart is hardened. The word that a hard "wayside" heart hears is immediately stolen by Satan.

When the word is planted on stony ground, it is compared to people who gladly hear and receive the word, but they have no room for roots to take hold.

When affliction or persecution arises for the word's sake, immediately they are offended.
Mark 4:17

These people did not take the time to learn the word for themselves and hide it in their hearts. They didn't understand the foundational principles of covenant. They may have expected an immediate manifestation and had no understanding that Satan was trying to steal the word from them. So they are offended by the word. These would be the people who say, "I tried "it" but "it" didn't work for me." They are the people only looking to receive signs and wonders and not a personal relationship with Jesus, who is the word made manifest.

The third example is when the word is sown among thorns.

The cares of this world and the deceitfulness of riches and the lust of other things entering in choke the word and it becomes unfruitful. Mark 4:19

To be honest, this is where most of us are. Even now some of you may be reading this word and get excited about understanding the healing power of Jesus provided for us at Calvary over 2000 years ago, but we let the busyness of our lives change our focus from the things of God. We get distracted by the reports from the doctors, the beliefs of our other Christian friends, and the medical bills piling up. Before we know it, the word, about which we were once so excited, gets choked, and does not produce the fruit for which we were looking in our lives. We begin to make decisions based on circumstances, rather than on direction from God. Like Peter (Matt. 14:28–31) who had the faith to get out of the boat in the middle of a storm and walk on the water to Jesus, we take our eyes off Jesus and on to that storm and we begin to sink.

Remember, there are two realities. One is the physical world; the world we can see and touch. The other is the spiritual realm. Sometimes we become so entrenched in the physical that it becomes difficult to remember God and see his reality. The world may have facts, but God's word is truth. We must step away from the cares of the world and return our focus on him.

There is a difference between faith and hope. Hope is for the future. Faith is now. It is not just a promise; it is a statement of fact. Faith sees the reality as already done. It sees what God sees.

When the word is sown on good ground, people hear the word, understand it, and receive it as fact. That word then brings the desired fruit, "some thirtyfold, some sixty, and some one hundred" (Mark 4:20).

> **But without faith it is impossible to please him, for he that comes to God must believe that he is and that he is a rewarder of them that diligently seek him. Hebrews 11:6**

Some people interpret this to mean we have to work for our reward. Certainly God's grace and mercy are free gifts, but just like salvation you have to receive it. Our spirits are born again by grace alone, but the mind needs regeneration. God expects us to learn and grow, so that our souls are not kept in the carnal realm, but are spirit-minded. We need to constantly renew our minds to the word of God (Rom.12: 2) and be cleansed by the washing of water by the word (Eph. 5:26). Only then can we resist the attacks of the devil and stand on our faith in the promises of God.

Let's look carefully at the 22 examples cited.

- Three are demonic deliverances
- Three appear to be acts of grace to a person with an unknown or questionable spiritual state. Jesus had to later address their spiritual state.
- 16 people moved in faith in Jesus, the manifested word of God. They heard the word and obeyed it. They had to have corresponding action to their belief that they were healed. Only when they acted on their faith did they see the healing.

- Six of the 16 were commended by Jesus for their faith and he actually told them that it was their faith that had made them well.
- To the two gentiles, the centurion and the Syrophenician woman, he said the phrase, "According to your faith, be it unto you."

Remember that everywhere that Jesus went, he first taught the people. He went about teaching, preaching, and healing every sickness and disease.

And Jesus went about all the cities and villages, teaching in their synagogues, and preaching the gospel of the kingdom, and healing every sickness and every disease among the people. Matthew 9:35

Notice that Jesus used a variety of ways to heal. He laid his hands on some, for some he did something unusual like spitting, and to some he spoke to the illness or spirit causing it. Many times he just asked the person to believe him and go convinced that it was done. God is God and he doesn't have to follow our formula for healing. Let him be God.

The purpose of sharing these examples is to build your faith and to help you see that it is God's will to heal you. We have to understand the principles of God so that we do not depend on psyching ourselves up to believe. We need to come to the place where we know that we know that we know!

So shall my word be that goes forth out of my mouth; it shall not return to me void [empty] but it shall accomplish that which I please and it shall prosper in the thing whereto I sent it. Isaiah 55:11

CHAPTER FOUR

Hindrances to Divine Healing

Delayed healings

One of the greatest hindrances to faith for healing comes when the immediate manifestation we were expecting is not seen and the healing requires us to stand in faith no matter how circumstances may look.

When I was in my twenties, I worked with an evangelist, who was anointed to pray for the sick. We saw many miraculous healings, but the teaching was limited. Unfortunately, frequently the same people would be back in the prayer line within a few weeks. They did not understand about what the word teaches about healing. They thought they needed an external touch and always looked for signs and wonders or they could not believe.

Listen to these life changing words from E.W. Kenyon in his book *Jesus the Healer*.

> **For many years I have been bothered because I could not understand why people, who had received their healing and had all the evidences of perfect deliverance, should have the diseases return. I believe I have made the discovery. Their faith was not in the word of God, but in "sense evidence." What do I mean by sense evidence?**

I mean the evidence of their sight, hearing and feeling...Many have no time to be taught the word. They have no interest in the Bible. They have no desire for the word. All they want is a healing-deliverance for themselves...It lies in this: They had no faith in the word of God. They knew nothing about the word, as far as healing is concerned. Their faith was in me, or in some other person, not in God's word. The Bible declares: By his stripes, I am healed.

(Osborn, p. 173)

I saw a man in a wheelchair come forward in a service where a minister planned to pray for the sick. This man was anointed with oil, prayed over, and then was wheeled back to his seat. He did not act on his faith and so did not see the "evidence" of healing. He thought healing was not for him. He did not have faith in the word of God and did not plan to take the time to understand it. He looked for a minister to believe for him. Certainly there are wonderful miracles as the Spirit wills, but God is looking for faith in people who call themselves Christians.

Another great man of God, Rev. Norval Hayes, was holding services in our church. After teaching about healing, he told the people that he would not lay hands of the sick. Laying on of hands is a foundational principle of the Bible (Heb. 6:2), but Norval said God showed him that the people were looking to him for the healing instead of Jesus. He added that anyone who wanted to come forward to receive a healing should come and kneel down at the altar and believe they receive. Some left disappointed that day, but some were touched by Jesus.

Delays in seeing our healing can work to make positive changes in us if we let them. For one, our pride and self-sufficiency is broken down. We recognize that we cannot get through this experience without God and so we begin to seek Him more diligently. He becomes a part of our every thought and action. Things of the world, like pleasures and distractions, fall away as irrelevant.

When our daughter Gabrielle received her diagnosis of lymphoma, I sat with her as the doctor explained that the PET scan showed that the cancer filled her neck and there were secondary spots in her spleen and right hip. The doctor recommended chemotherapy and possibly radiation to begin immediately. We went in to that office full of the word of God. Gabrielle smiled at the doctor and told her that she appreciated everything that the doctor would do for her, but that Jesus was her healer.

While my husband and I would have preferred no treatment, Gabrielle at twenty-eight-years-old was an adult and had to make her own decision. She decided to allow six months of chemotherapy with four hours every two weeks. I was with her when the chemotherapy port was surgically put into her chest and tried to come to as many of the chemo sessions as possible. She never complained of having any of the side effects of chemo and remained cheerful and full of faith during those times.

One night during that first week while sleeping in her living room, I got up with a strong urge to pray. I walked around that apartment praying in the spirit, and stood outside the door of her bedroom laying my hands on the door and praying. In the morning I learned that Gabrielle was also awake during the night. The pain in her right hip had become so strong that she could not sleep. She walked around that room saying, "Oh no you don't Satan. I am healed by the blood of Jesus. You take your hands off me."

My whole family immersed ourselves in the word. In Florida, my son Mike sent his sister daily reminders of the promises of God and exhortations of faith. In Connecticut, my daughter Mary and her husband Chris agreed in the prayer of faith. In Virginia, Gabrielle and her roommate filled the apartment with scriptures pasted on every cabinet door, mirror, and any available space. We refused to confess anything except what Jesus said.

Delays show us where we are really located with God. Does what we say we believe really stand up in a time of testing? God wants to heal us, but more importantly, he wants to mold us in his image. In the end, the condition of our spirit is more important to him than our circumstances. He wants us to see with our spiritual eyes instead of our fleshly ones. He wants us to grow in our understanding of the Word.

Delays stretch our faith and make us strong and assured, as we draw close to the presence of God. Nehemiah 8:10 says, "The joy of the Lord is our strength." We learn the great release there is in praising him.

> **Therefore I take pleasure in infirmities [sickness and disease], in reproaches [insults], in necessities, in persecutions, in distresses for Christ's sake: for when I am weak, then am I strong.**
> **II Corinthians 2:10**

This may seem ridiculous in the eyes of the world. Maybe that is where the reproaches come into the picture. Some people might even use this verse to say, "I'm suffering for the Jesus." They miss the end of the verse that says that we are strong because we are dependent, not on our own strength, but on his.

> **I can do all things through Christ that strengthens me. Philippians 4:13**

His strength can do all things. Nothing is impossible to him. That is why we can "take pleasure in sicknesses". We know Christ is our healer. We can jump and leap for joy over that knowledge.

As we wait on the Lord, we find peace that passes understanding, joy unspeakable, and a deeper love for God and each other. Delays develop the precious fruit of the spirit in our lives (Gal. 5:22–23).

We can wait in full assurance that God already provided our healing with Jesus's broken body. God hears and answers prayer.

During this time of waiting for the physical manifestation of the healing, we have to be prepared for spiritual warfare. We have to wear the full armor of God to stand against the wiles of the devil (Eph. 6:10-18). We must be prepared to "Fight the good fight of faith" (I Tim. 6:12). Know your enemy has been defeated by Jesus and know we are "more than conquerors through him that loved us" (Rom. 8:37).

After two months, Gabrielle had a second PET. I personally saw both scans. The second scan showed no spots of cancer anywhere in Gabrielle's body. We wanted them to immediately stop chemotherapy, but they refused due to some insurance regulations and liability concerns. We then had to pray that no deadly things would harm her! After six months, Gabrielle insisted that the chemotherapy port be removed and it was. She has not had any further treatment although she has to keep returning for PET scans to confirm the cancer is gone. Now her sweet doctor asks to hug her when she comes for appointments. The doctor recognizes that she has witnessed a miracle, which she calls "fantastical results." Looking back, our regret is that we did not demand a second PET scan immediately after the original one, because God's healing had occurred as soon as we prayed! We just needed the corresponding faith action! Thank God, we are growing and learning and he is patient with us.

Watch your mouth

The Book of James has a lot to say about the tongue and the difficulty to control it.

> **And the tongue is a fire, a world of iniquity, so is the tongue among our members, that it defiles the whole body and sets on fire the course of nature and it is set on fire of hell. James 3:6**

And in Proverbs of Solomon,

> **Death and life are in the power of the tongue
> and they that love it shall eat the fruit thereof.
> Proverbs 18:21**

We say we believe God for healing, but the words that come out of our mouths speak fear, disbelief, and confusion. The opposite of faith.

> **Even so faith, if it has not works, is dead, being
> alone...I will show you my faith by my works.
> James 2:17,18b**

Works is not a dirty word. It just means that if you truly believe something, then it will change your actions. Do we really understand the importance of our words? Our words locate our heart's position.

> **But those things which proceed out of the mouth
> come forth from the heart, and they defile the
> man. Matthew 15:18**

> **We having the same spirit of faith, according
> as it is written, I believed, and therefore I have
> spoken; we also believe, and therefore speak. II
> Corinthians 4:13**

Hebrews 11:1 teaches us that faith is a *substance* [the concrete essence, confidence] of things we are hoping for and it is the *evidence* [proof] of things we have not yet seen. If you have prayed and believed to receive something in the will of God (and you are convinced as I am that healing is the will of God), then the word says, "He shall have whosoever he saith" (Mark 11:23).

Mediate on this until it become real to you. If you know that you have something, even if it hasn't materialized, you have it.

When I start a job and the boss says that I will receive my paycheck at the end of the week, I believe him, and do my job, even without the evidence of the money in my hand. I know that it is coming. How can we can have faith in a flawed, earthly boss, but doubt the word of our gracious, eternal Father?

A child who is promised that the parent has a gift for him after school will be joyful all day. That is how we should be reacting. We should be full of joy and singing praises to our God for the answered prayer. We would be shouting "I'm healed!"

Instead, people pray, say they believe God, and then often get on the phone and cry to others about the problem. Or they get off their knees and repeat what the doctor has said about their condition instead of what Jesus assures us is the truth.

I remember watching a wonderful elderly English minister pray for the sick. A woman came for healing for a bad back. The minister prayed and then said, "Now touch your toes." Her response was, "I can't. I have a bad back." The minister shook his head and told her to go sit down. The woman went away as she had come, unhealed.

T.L. Osborn tells a wonderful story of a daughter sick with tuberculosis that learned in the word of God that by his strips she was healed. She excitedly told her mother and asked her mother if she believed it too. The mother said yes, but then was horrified when the daughter wanted to put on her clothes and get out of bed. The mother, who said she believed, tried to persuade her to stay in bed. The daughter insisted that healed people do not stay in bed. Thank God, she got up and dressed herself and went around the house shouting praises to God. She was completely healed and restored in less than three weeks. [Osborn, page 69]

Do you see the faith in this girl's works? She believed for her deliverance with her heart and so it was the most natural thing for her to speak it with her mouth and do the corresponding actions.

The mother said she believed, but her corresponding words and actions were not there.

For with the heart, man believes unto righteousness and with the mouth, confession is made unto salvation [deliverance, health, safety, salvation]. Romans 10:10

Novel Hayes told us a story about his daughter who had deformed hands. As a Baptist, he got hold of teachings on healing and so prayed for the healing of his daughter's hands. The hands remained unchanged, but every day he thanked God for her healing. She would get frustrated and tell him, "Dad, I'm not healed!" He said he was not moved by anything but the word of God. One day, while putting a box up on a shelf, she screamed. Her hands were completely restored.

I know what I am saying is not always easy. It is frequently a fight. We have an enemy who wants to fill you fear and doubts. Do not fight Satan's thoughts with your own thoughts. When we pray, find scriptures to stand on, and feel convinced. Then we need to resist any thought contrary to that Jesus has said. Thank God I am learning what to do with the unbelief coming out of my mouth. I tell my carnal mouth to shut up! I renew my mind with the word of God, until my spirit and mind are in agreement and says what God says. Like Jesus, we boldly say, "It is written!"

One of my favorite verses is found in II Corinthians 10:3–6.

For though we walk in the flesh, we do not war after the flesh; For the weapons of our warfare are not carnal, but mighty through God to the pulling down of strongholds; Casting down imaginations and every high thing that exalteth itself against the knowledge of God, and bringing into captivity every thought to the obedience

of Christ; and having a readiness to revenge all disobedience when your obedience is fulfilled.

This takes a disciplined life of bringing the mind and body under the authority of the spirit. The understood noun here is YOU. You cast down imaginations and anything that tries to raise itself higher than the word of God. You bring every thought to obedience of Christ. You get ready to revenge all disobedience to that word. You control that fiery tongue that sets the course of nature. Say what Jesus says or say nothing!

And I know that His commandment is life everlasting: whatsoever I speak therefore even as the Father said unto me, so I speak. John 12:50

Sudden Attacks

Some attacks happen before we can know or understand what has happened, like an auto accident or sudden sickness or collapse. Sometimes doctors shock you with a diagnosis and will try to persuade you to make an immediate decision, such as surgery, before you have time to feed your spirit and hear specific directions from God. A life-altering decision might be made that would never have been made under normal circumstances.

I know this is what happened to Gabrielle. The doctor stressed the importance of taking immediate action. There was no time to waste. Thank God, Gabrielle had spent the last few days meditating on the word. She told the concerned doctor that she had upcoming plans for a few weeks that she would not change. She refused to feel rushed or pressured into making her decision for treatment as if her life depended on that treatment rather than on God. Only when she felt assured in her own spirit did she start treatment.

I am learning in my own life, when faced with a crisis or emergency, my first response must be automatic. I must talk to Jesus first. I go to my "garden spot" and wait until I hear from him. He gives the peace that passes understanding (Phil. 4:7) and the mind of Christ (1 Cor. 2:16) to know what to do.

For we walk by faith, not by sight.
II Corinthians 5:7

Sometimes the very nature of the illness causes the person to feel weak and vulnerable. Possibly it is hard for that person to function. In these cases they may have to depend on the decision of a loved one whose ultimate goal is moved by love and possibly fear of losing the person they hold so dear. They may move on emotion and human reasoning. It is hard to make a life or death decision for someone else.

Brother Kenneth Hagen told of a time that his wife was facing an illness and the doctors recommended surgery. He asked her for what she could believe God and she answered that she could believe for a successful surgery. He then agreed with her for that end. The surgery was a success and she was able to believe God for recovery. We need to agree with a person at the level of their faith and understanding.

The doctors once told me that they had found a suspicious lump and that I "might" have breast cancer. They wanted to schedule a biopsy and possible removal of any tumor they might find. Much to their surprise and consternation, I said no. As a nurse, I know how that works. If they find the lump is cancerous, they would want to continue the procedure to eradicate the cancer and possibly my breast while I was under anesthesia.

After discussing the situation with my husband, I stated that if I did have cancer, I would believe God for healing. It seemed that the smartest thing to do was to believe God for his removal of the lump whether it was cancerous or not. We agreed together in prayer and forgot about it. After six months, an upset doctor asked me at least to re-take the scan and examination. I did so in faith and no lumps were found.

Medical professionals want to make you well, but they frequently do not have the mind of Christ and generally depend on the wisdom of man rather than God. Much of their work may be trial and error and experimentation. I am frustrated with their need to keep "doing everything they can do", even when they know there is no hope in the natural. They surgically cut people, subject them to medications and treatments that weaken the person's own ability to fight disease, and usually destroy the person's quality of life and desire to live. They do this, not to be unkind, but rather in their sincere desire to help and to use their learning. They often put undue pressure and guilt on the person and family.

I am not belittling the work of medicine. God has inspired men and women to do great things through it. Numerous wonderful medical advances have been made. Man does his best, but still is fallible and limited. God is not. We must never allow medical science to be believed and relied upon over God himself. Remember, science is the study of what God already knows!

If someone, maybe yourself, has been a person taken by surprise by a sudden illness, you can start to believe him for healing where you are located now. It will be a valiant fight of faith and may even require a time when you will need to tell the doctors and your loved ones "enough!" Remember the woman with the issue of blood who for 12 years was treated by doctors and only got worse? She finally knew that her only answer was in Jesus Christ.

Whatever your decision is, make sure your direction comes from God. Then you can go forward in full assurance whatever the course you take.

When he, the Spirit of truth, is come, he will guide you into all truth: for he shall not speak of himself, but whatsoever he shall hear, that shall he speak, and he will show you things to come. John 16:13

Out of Covenant Relationship

Another hindrance to receiving your healing is when we forget our covenant relationship and have unaddressed sin issues in our lives. These issues are dangerous because they hinder our ability to believe God with a pure heart.

The Bible clearly tells us that God is good, merciful, longsuffering, and gracious. He does not sit in heaven waiting for someone to goof up so he can take out his big whip. He does not discipline his children by throwing them down a staircase or putting their hands on a hot fire. James called God "The Father of Lights" and incapable to doing evil. He is the God described in Psalms 103,

Who forgiveth all thine iniquities and who healeth all thy diseases; who redeemeth thy life from destruction, who crowneth thee with loving-kindness and tender mercies; who satisfieth thy mouth with good things, so that thy youth is renewed like the eagle's. (v. 3-5)

After a wonderful list of blessings afforded to God's children, the Psalmist adds,

To such as keep his covenant, and to those that remember his commandments to do them. (v. 18)

People like to say that we are all children of God. But that isn't true, is it? We live in an age where "tolerance" and "acceptance" are esteemed; where right and wrong is "relative" and where people are told to live true to their own beliefs. Christians that do not conform to these views are labeled ignorant, narrow-minded, bigoted, and judgmental.

God has not changed. We live in a time of great grace in the body of Christ. However, God still has a standard of holiness and tells us to be holy, as he is holy. His reaction to sin and disobedience has not changed. He still will judge sin. I do not believe that means he will give you sickness. It does mean that you have to may go through things of your own making.

How do we reconcile these two different pictures of God? One is loving and merciful and the other is the jealous God who punishes sin. We have all failed and God knows our weaknesses, but when we get out from underneath the covering of his protection and covenant, we expose ourselves to all the evil in the world.

Let me give you an example from my own life. In college I had felt the call of God on my life, but after graduating, circumstances caused me to be focused on getting a job and supporting myself. I started dating a very nice man, but a man who did not share the same beliefs in God as I did. I was hearing the voice of God in the back of my mind and knew something was wrong in my life, but ignored the warnings. One evening as I was returning from the man's home, my car spun on ice until it crashed. The car was totaled and I had some broken bones and pain. Did God cause that accident to punish me? No. I was in the wrong place. Could God have prevented the accident? Yes. I am sure through the years God has protected me from many other accidents. It was not God's choice for me to be removed from covenant protection; it was mine. I was the one not listening to the warnings and was not obedient to his word.

I love the words of Psalms 139. I hope that you will take the time to carefully and prayerfully read the entire chapter. Listen to the final words:

Search me, oh God, and know my heart: try me and know my thoughts: And see if there be any wicked way in me, and lead me in the way everlasting. (v. 23, 24)

Each of us must take the time to ask the Lord to search our hearts. Have I opened the door for this attack from Satan because

I have lost my first love and strayed from my closeness to the Lord? Have I harbored hatred and unforgiveness in my heart? Are there things that I need to make right in my walk with the Lord? Am I in the wrong place at the wrong time and with the wrong people? Do I find it hard now to believe God for help and deliverance? A person who does not feel the need to judge and correct themselves has displayed a heart that is not soft and pliable before the Lord.

Please understand that attacks from Satan can be the result of being exactly where we should be. A Vietnam War pilot once told me that the way you know you are over enemy territory is when someone is firing back at you! Satan just wants to stop us from serving the Lord! Sometimes we are innocently suffering from the effects of a fallen world with pestilence, pollution, and contamination. You alone will be able to answer the sin question in your own life.

Jesus knew these things would be confusing at times to us. He understood that we live in a fallen, corrupt world where bad things happen to good people and bad people alike. In the natural, we just do not know all the factors that might cause diseases like cancer. Instead of over-spiritualizing every event, he told us to look to the most important issue of our relationship to God and eternity.

Or those eighteen, upon whom the tower in Siloam fell, and slew them; think ye that they were sinners above all men that dwelt in Jerusalem? I tell you, Nay; but except ye repent ye shall all likewise perish. Luke 13:4, 5

If Jesus waited for us to be perfect before we could receive from him, none of us would be able to believe to receive salvation or healing. While the Holy Spirit convicts of sin, Satan brings condemnation and shame. Believing that you are not good enough to receive a healing is putting the focus on you, instead of where it belongs; Jesus and his redeeming grace!

The good news is that God always provides a remedy and a way of escape. Ask him to forgive you! He will and the angels will rejoice over your decision.

> **Beloved, if our heart condemn us not, than have we confidence toward God. And whatsoever we ask, we receive of him, because we keep his commandments, and do those things that are pleasing in his sight. I John 3:21, 22**

Unhealthy Lifestyles

While not necessarily sin, we often neglect to listen to God about what is necessary for a healthy lifestyle. It is important that we listen to the voice of the Lord about how we live our lives. So many diseases are preventable even in the medical world. Has God been speaking to you about the foods you eat, what you drink, and your need for exercise? Probably stress and lack of rest are two of the greatest causes of strain on your heart and entire system. All of these are dealt with in the word of God.

I used to tell my students that I believe God in his goodness has all the cures we need right here on earth, even the cure for cancer, in herbs and plants. Certainly the old timers like my father-in-law, a Canadian back woods man, knew something about this. He knew that a pretty, little yellow plant grew beside poison ivy and could be grounded into the antidote for the poisonous plant. He knew that the extract from certain tree barks could fight infections. The list could go on and on.

I know of many people who knew that they must stop a certain damaging lifestyle such as junk food, gluttony, sodas, cigarettes, alcohol, drugs, or promiscuous sex and ignored the warnings and died. Possibly they were caught in the web of addiction and didn't know how to escape. God's Old Testament laws are still wise life practices and still work when applied sensibly. The New Testament shows us how to defeat the enemy of addiction by being filled with the Spirit of God and the word of God.

We must make God a part of every aspect of our lives. Listen intently to him and obey him. Remember that while God has provided guidelines to follow, he is still our healer no matter what mistakes we may have made in caring for ourselves in the past or what external forces attack us now. Believe for your healing. Then start taking care of your body for the glory of God!

Stinking Thinking

Most of our difficulties in receiving healing come from poor teaching in the church world. We have not been taught that both salvation and healing were provided by the death and resurrection of Jesus Christ.

In summary, I have listed several areas that we need to check ourselves to see if we have "stinking thinking" and do not understand or believe the word. Ask yourself these questions.

1. Do you believe that Jesus provided both your salvation and your healing by his blood and broken body?
2. Do you believe that healing is always the will of God? God is not a respecter of persons. Jesus came to give you abundant life. He wants you healed.
3. Do you understand that Satan is your enemy not God? Once you believe that Satan gave you the illness and not God, you will be able to fight Satan as Jesus did when he said, "It is written."
4. Do you know the Word of God as it pertains to healing or do you refuse to search it out?

"Faith comes by hearing and hearing the word of God." (Rom. 10:17)

5. Do you want a "drive-through" healing, a fast miracle, and not the miracle worker? Jesus explained why he spoke in parables. He wanted people to desire, search and dig for truth. He said, "Therefore I speak to them in parables, because they seeing, see not and hearing, they hear not, neither do they understand." (Matt. 13:13)

6. Do you believe or understand that there will be things that God wants you to do? "Go wash in the pool", "Go show yourself to priest", "Pick up your bed", "Stretch forth your hand". The list goes on and on.

7. Do you understand that your words have power over life and death? Are you saying what Jesus says about your situation? (Prov. 18:21)

8. Do you have corresponding actions to what you say you are believing?

"But will you know, O vain man, that faith without works is dead?" (James 2:20)

9. Do you see yourself as healed, restored, strong and full of life or can you not picture what a healed self would look like?

10. Do you understand that you will never be "good enough" to receive healing, any more than you were "good enough" to be saved? It is God's goodness, not yours.

11. Do you recognize that Christ is in you and his strength is yours?

"If the Spirit of him that raised up Jesus from the dead dwell in you, he that raised up Christ from the dead shall also quicken [give life] your moral bodies by his Spirit that dwells in you." (Rom. 8:11)

12. Do you treat your body like the holy temple where God lives? (II Cor. 6:19)

13. Do you live a life full of praise and joy and peace, thanking God for what he has given you now and what he will give you in the future?

Rejoice in the Lord always: and again I say rejoice. Let your moderation [patience] be known unto all men. The Lord is at hand [near and ready]. Be careful [having anxious thought] for nothing, but in everything by prayer and supplication [requests] with thanksgiving [thankfulness as an act of worship] let your requests be made known unto God. And the peace of God, which passeth all understanding, shall keep your hearts and minds through Christ Jesus. Philippians 4:4–7

Chapter Five
The Meaning in Communion

As we carefully studied the word of God, we saw a new depth of meaning in communion as shown by Jesus in the last supper. At the time of the last supper, Jesus had not gone to the cross yet, and so the disciples did not fully understand the significance of his words or actions.

Today many of his modern day disciples still do not understand. Later Paul had a deeper revelation about the significance of communion in I Corinthians 11:24–25, 27–30. The passage is from King James, but Strong's concordance definition is in brackets. Take some time and think about this passage.

> **And when he had given thanks, he brake it and said, Take eat: this is my body which is broken for you: this do in remembrance of me. And after the same manner also he took the cup, when he had supped saying, This cup is the new testament [covenant] in my blood: This do ye as oft as ye drink it in remembrance of me.**
>
> **Therefore whosoever shall eat this bread, and drink this cup of the Lord unworthily [impudently, irreverently], shall be guilty [bound, liable, under obligation] of the body and blood of the Lord.**

But let a man examine himself, and so let him eat of that bread, and drink of that cup. For he that eateth and drinketh unworthily, eateth and drinketh damnation [condemnation] to himself, not discerning the Lord's body. For this cause many are weak and sickly among you and many sleep.

The word discerning can be interpreted in many ways. The definitions include "making a distinction between", "discriminating", "giving judgment" and "separating". Greek scholars say "properly distinguishing". So the verse could read "eats and drinks condemnation to himself, not making a properly distinction concerning the Lord's body.

All churchgoers have heard these words or some part of them. Growing up in the Protestant church, I took communion the first Sunday of every month. It was a time to reflect on my life, repent for sins, and thank God for his mercy. I thought, as most Christians, that it was solely ordained by Jesus as a way to remember him. I also thought that if I had any sin when I took communion, God would punish me and I could get sick or die! No one ever explained to me the error in that thinking.

There is so much more here to understand and appreciate. Jesus at the last supper took the bread, gave thanks, and broke it. Then he gave it to the disciples telling them that it represented his body which was broken for them. He exhorted them to remember him when they took it. He later told them to take the cup which represented his blood that he was going to shed for them.

The church has no problem understanding the cup. We understand that Jesus had to go to Calvary to have his blood shed for the forgiveness of sin and, as High Priest, to apply that blood to the mercy seat (Heb. 2:17; 4:14–16).

Up until the time of Jesus, the blood of animals had to be offered yearly by the earthly priest for the cleansing of a person's sins. At the time of Moses and the exodus from Egypt, every Israelite who put the lamb's blood over their doorposts were saved from the devastation coming to the Egyptians.

Throughout the Bible we see that covenants were made with the shedding of blood, starting with God killing an animal to cover the nakedness of Adam and Eve to Jesus' ultimate sacrifice for sin.

And almost all things are by the law purged with blood and without shedding of blood is no remission [pardon, letting sins go as if they were never committed]…now once in the end of the world has he appeared to put away sin by the sacrifice of himself. (Hebrews 9:22, 26b)

Much more then, being now justified [regarded as innocent] by his blood, we shall be saved from the wrath through him. Romans 5:9

So when we take the cup at communion, we are acknowledging the full or complete sacrifice that our God made for us in order to have forgiveness of our sins. We are exhorted to take this cup reverently, with a repentant, thankful, loving heart toward God for his unspeakable mercy to us.

We understand about the blood but what about the body? When the Israelites were instructed to kill a spotless lamb and apply the blood to the doorposts, what happened to the body of the lamb? The Israelites were instructed to eat the lamb's flesh for strength and health for their journey to the promise land.

I had a nutrition teacher in college who often said, "You are what you eat." This is true because normally the body breaks down what you eat into the nutrients you need for life. Jesus told us to take the bread as a symbol of his body and eat it in remembrance of him. Well, what do we remember about his body? It was bruised and whipped for us. But for what purpose? Why couldn't he simply have his throat cut like the Old Testament lambs, if all that was needed was his blood to be shed? Isaiah prophesied in Isaiah 53:5

> **But he was wounded for our transgressions [sins, rebellion], he was bruised [beat to pieces] for our iniquities [moral evil, sin]; and the chastisement [correction, discipline] of our peace [safety, welfare, favor] was upon him and with his stripes [bruises, wounds] we are healed [cured as by a physician, made whole].**

God gave the Apostle Matthew a sovereign revelation about what Isaiah saw in prophesy and explained even further:

> **That it might be fulfilled which was spoken by Esaias the prophet saying, Himself took our infirmities [sicknesses, diseases] and bore our sicknesses [diseases, infirmities]. Matthew 8:17**

Both salvation and healing are equally part of the redemption provided at Calvary. Satan comes to steal, kill, and destroy (John 10:10), but Jesus came to give us abundant life. Satan does not want us to know that God planned for our healing of sicknesses, just as he planned for our salvation from sin. Sickness should have no more power over us than sin does. David said in Psalms 103:2–3,

> **Bless the Lord, Oh my soul, and forget not all his benefits. Who forgives all your iniquities [sins] and who heals all your diseases [sicknesses].**

When we take the bread at communion, we are to remember the body of Christ. When we eat the bread, we remember that we have the life of Christ inside of us and Christ's life flows through us giving us strength and health. We remember that because of his stripes, we were healed (I Peter 2:24).

Now look again at the conclusion of Paul's explanation of communion.

> **But let a man examine himself, and so let him eat of that bread and drink of that cup. For he that eats and drinks unworthily, eateth and drinketh damnation [condemnation] to himself, not discerning [thoroughly separating, judging] the Lord's body. For this cause many are weak and sickly among you and many sleep. I Corinthians 11:28–30**

It was like a light bulb went off and we could see clearly what God was saying to us. We always understood that the Lord's blood was shed for our sin and by it we can receive forgiveness and cleansing. The problem is most churches stop there. They do not discern the Lord's body.

We need to make the distinction about the body which was brutally broken for us. Jesus said we were to partake of the bread in remembrance of Him. Jesus told us, "Do this in remembrance of me."

If we do not rightly divide the word of God and understand that his body was broken and wounded for our healing, and that healing is the children's bread as Jesus explained, we can remain sickly and even die in our sickness.

Now when we take communion, it always has special significance to us. We remember all that Jesus did for us on that blessed Passover. His blood was applied for the forgiveness of our sins. His body was broken for our healing. The sacrifice of the blood and the body continue to be available to all who believe in them. Salvation and healing were both provided for us by the Father through the Son!

CHAPTER SIX

God Yearns To Heal You

I love the word yearns. The Cambridge dictionary defines it as to desire something strongly, especially something difficult or impossible to obtain. The Old English definition includes the meaning to be filled with compassion and warm feelings of deep affection.

In church we extol the great power of God. We pray for greater manifestation of that power. It seems that having that power demonstrated helps us know that he is near and cares about what happens in our lives.

Even the Devil knows God is powerful and able to heal. What he tries to keep people from knowing is the depth of God's compassion for us. Our God is a merciful God.

> **O give thanks unto the Lord for he is good [bountiful, gracious, kind] and his mercy [favor, kindness] endures forever. I Chronicles 16:34**

F.F. Bosworth once said that it is not about knowing what God *can* do that builds faith. It is what he *yearns to do.*

God wants everyone to be saved from his or her sins, but he cannot violate his own laws of free will. Healing too is a free gift and has to be accepted with faith in a loving Father. Jesus showed us the heart of God when he moved in compassion for the masses of hurt and sick people. He longs to touch and heal.

Jesus taught his disciples to pray, God's will be done on earth as it is in heaven. Well, praise God, there is no sickness in heaven!

Thy kingdom come. Thy will be done in earth as it is in heaven. Matthew 6:10

God is good… all the time. He yearns to pour out his blessing on his children.

The eyes of the Lord run to and fro throughout the whole earth to show himself strong [strengthen, cure, help, and repair] in behalf of them whose heart is perfect [complete, peaceable, ready] toward him.

II Chronicles. 16:9

Can you picture that? God is looking throughout the world for people that are ready, willing, and eager for his great mercy. Strong's concordance states that "running to and fro" can be explained as a mariner lashing through the seas with oars. God is running his eyes over this earth looking for you! Our great God longs to be good, but we have to get people to hear and seek the Lord.

In my younger days, I was excitedly just learning about the spirit realm and the power in prayer. One day, I was loudly praying up a storm over urgent needs, when it was if a loud voice yelled in my ear, "I heard you!" It was so real and strong, that I immediately stopped and began laughing. God got his point across to me. We don't need to shout or plead or whine. We don't have to make deals. God hears us and wants to answer with his love and mercy.

I have learned that while it may be easy to pray, there comes a time when we have to get up and believe. Knowing that the One that I am talking to loves me and wants only my best, changes the whole dynamic of prayer. I am speaking to my heavenly father and he loves me. We are in an intimate relationship.

> **That he would grant you, according to the riches of *his* glory, to be strengthened with might by *his* Spirit in the inner man; That Christ may dwell in your hearts by faith, that ye being *rooted and grounded in love,* may be able to comprehend with all saints what is the breadth and length and depth and height, and to know the *love of Christ, with passeth knowledge,* that ye might be filled with all the fullness of God. Now unto *him* that is able to do exceeding *abundantly above* all that we ask or think, according to the power that works in us. (Italic is my emphasis). Ephesians 3:16–20**

Do you notice that it is his glory, his spirit, his love? This love passes all human understanding. Do not put the focus on you. He is the one who loves you and it is his power working in you. Rooted and grounded in love! What life changing words.

Listen to these popular verses with a heart eager to know your heavenly Father better.

> **And I say unto you, Ask, and it shall be given you; seek, and ye shall find; knock, and it shall be opened to you. For everyone that asketh receiveth; and he that seeketh findeth, and to him that knocketh it shall be opened. If a son shall ask bread of any of you that is a father, will he give him a stone? Or if he ask a fish will he for a fish give him a serpent? Or if he shall ask an egg, will he offer him a scorpion? If ye then, being evil, know how to give good gifts**

unto your children, how much more shall your heavenly Father give the Holy Spirit to them that ask him? (Luke 11: 9–13)

F.F. Bosworth said, "It seems to me that God would rather we doubt his power, than his willingness."

When I was in my 20's, a friend of my sister's was diagnosed with a cancerous tumor in her brain. She had tried for many years to have a child and while delivering her little girl, the brain tumor was discovered. The doctors did not give her hope. I went alone to my room to pray, but instead I began to tell God off for his unfairness to this sweet Christian family. In midst of my tears and anger, I heard that still, strong voice change the direction of my thoughts and tell me to read Psalms 147:11. That is a rather obscure verse and I had no idea what it said, so opened to it immediately. It read,

The Lord takes pleasure in them that fear him, in those that hope in his mercy.

My own paraphrased English puts it this way:

It makes God happy when he finds people who will trust him and expect him to be kind and good.

I immediately understood what God was telling me. It gives him joy when we believe he is a good, merciful, and loving Father. It shows we know him! I wrote to this friend immediately sharing what God had said to me. She later told me that, when she opened to that scripture, she felt the presence of God. She called her husband and he had the same experience. They made God happy that day by believing in his great love. She and her husband went on to become grandparents!

Doesn't it seem to be an insult when we question the very character and nature of God?

The Bible is full of verses about God's love and mercy. Mediate on them until they take root in your heart.

He delights in mercy. Micah 7:18

Hear me, oh Lord, for thy loving-kindness is good; turn to me according to the multitude of your tender mercies. Psalms 69:16

The Lord is good to all; and his tender mercies are over all his works. Psalms 145:9

I will sing of the mercies of the Lord forever; with my mouth will I make known your faithfulness to all generations. Psalms 89:1

Like a Father pities [love, compassionate] his children, so the Lord pities them that fear [reverence] him. Psalms 103:13

But the mercy of the Lord is from everlasting to everlasting upon them that fear him and his righteousness unto children's children. Psalms 103:17

And said, O Lord God of Israel, there is no God like you in the heaven nor in the earth, which keeps covenant and shows mercy unto your servants that walk before you with all their hearts.
II Chronicles 6:14

Blessed be God, even the Father of our Lord Jesus Christ, the Father of mercies and the God of all comfort. II Corinthians 1:3

He that spared not his own Son, but delivered him up for us all, how shall he not also freely give us all things? Romans 8:32

The Israelites recurrent song was, "The Lord is good and his mercies endures forever." Jesus said he came to show the works of the Father. Our Father is good and his mercies endure forever! God loves me and yearns to be good to me and my children and children's children. What a great God we serve!

T.L. Osborn said, "God's word becomes simple when we regard every word as true and act accordingly." (P.43)

When James gave instructions to the church, he said by the Holy Spirit,

Is there any sick among you? Let him call for the elders of the church and let them pray over him, anointing him with oil in the name of the Lord. And the prayer of faith shall save [deliver, heal, make whole] the sick. James 5:14–15a

Believing becomes as natural as breathing, when we put our faith in a God that loves us and wants us well. We do not have to conjure up something dramatic. He sent his only begotten Son to be bruised and beaten so we could have that healing.

He that spared not his own Son, but delivered him up for us all, how shall he not with him also freely give us all things? Romans 8:32

Remember, God yearns to heal you!

78

Chapter Seven

Your daily "Gospel-pills"

In those first days and weeks after Gabrielle's diagnosis, I searched The Word for scriptures on faith and healing and compiled the following list. It is in no way exhaustive. On the list I wrote the prescription to Gabrielle: take twice a day and as needed. It is impossible to over-dose on them! I took the liberty to put in the personal pronouns "I" and "Me". You can put your own name into the scripture as you speak it, because it's a promise for you. I pray you will use the prescription too.

> **By his stripes, I am healed. (I Peter 2:24)**
>
> **He heals all my diseases. (Ps. 103:3)**
>
> **Christ himself took my infirmities and bore my sickness. (Matt. 8:27)**
>
> **The Lord is the strength of my life, of whom shall I be afraid? (Ps. 27:1)**
>
> **Greater is He that is in me, than he that is in the world [my cancer]. (I John 4:4)**

God has delivered me from the power of darkness. (Col. 1:13)

I fear not because he is with me; I am not dismayed for my God will strengthen me and will help me. (Is. 41:10)

I can do all things through Christ who strengthens me. (Phil. 4:13)

I hold fast the confession of my faith without wavering for he is faithful that promised. (Heb. 10:23)

I am redeemed from the curse of the law [sickness] because Christ was made a curse for me. (Gal. 3:13)

I am bought with a price; therefore, I glorify God in my body and in my spirit which are the Lord God's. (I Cor. 6:20)

I am more than a conqueror through Him who loves me. (Rom. 8:37)

God is the God who heals me. (Ex. 15:26)

Jesus the son of God was manifested that he might destroy the works of the devil [this cancer]. (1 John 3:8)

I am his workmanship created in Christ Jesus. (Eph. 2:10)

I believe, therefore all things are possible. (Mark 9:23)

Christ is in me, the hope of glory. In me is the full Godhead bodily. (Col. 1: 27)

In Jesus' name, I have all authority to cast out devils [and demons who bring disease]. (Mark 16: 27)

Jesus is The Word and he lives inside me. (John 1:1)

God supplies all of my needs according to his riches in heaven. (Phil. 4:19)

God sent his word [Jesus] and healed me. (Ps. 107:20)

God's divine power has given to me all things that pertain unto life. (Peter 1:13)

Jesus gave all power over the enemy and nothing by any means can hurt me. (Luke 10:19)

No weapon formed against me will prosper. (Is. 54: 17)

Let the weak say I am strong. (Joel 3:10)

I overcome by the blood of the Lamb and the word of my testimony. (Rev. 12:11)

Jesus is the same yesterday, today and forever. (Heb. 13:8)

And this is the confidence that I have: that if I ask anything according to his will, he hears me and if he hears me, then I know I have the request of him. (I John 5:14)

With long life, he satisfies me and shows me his salvation. (Ps. 91: 16)

But we walk by faith and not by sight. (II Cor. 5:7)

This affliction will never rise up again. (Naham 9:1)

God said, "My covenant will I not break nor alter the thing that has come out of my lips". (Ps. 89: 34)

I will live and not die and declare the works of the Lord. (Ps. 118:17)

He sends his word and heals me and rescued me from the pit and destruction. (Ps. 107:20)

I trust the Lord with all my heart and do not rely on my [or the doctor's] understanding. In all my ways, I will acknowledge him and he makes my paths smooth. (Prov. 3: 5–6)

My son [or daughter] attends to God's words, inclines their ears to God's sayings. They do let them depart from their eyes; they keep them in the midst of their hearts; for they are life unto them who find them and health to their flesh. (Prov. 4:20–22)

God's word will not fail. Not one word failed of any good thing which the Lord spoken to the house of Israel. All came to pass. (Josh. 21: 45)

God's will [healing] is working in me, for it is God who works in me, both to will and to do for his good pleasure. (Phil. 2:13)

Be it unto me according to thy word. (Luke 1:38)

The God who calls things which be not as though they are. (Rom. 4:17)

I am the Lord. I will speak and the word that I speak shall come to pass. (Ezek. 12:25)

Heaven and earth shall pass away, but my words shall not pass away. (Matt. 24:25)

What he [God] has promised, he is able to perform. (Rom. 4: 21)

And so he fed them by the integrity of his heart and guided them by the skillfulness of his hands. (Ps. 78: 72)

For all the promises of God in him are yea and in him amen, unto the glory of God by us. (II Cor. 1:20)

REMEMBER: If you don't let go of what you believe, then Satan has to!

Chapter Eight
Gabrielle's Story in Her Words

It never occurred to me that I would have to call my mom one morning to tell her I had cancer. I remember those moments between the calls with my doctor and my mom. So many thoughts at once. So many fears. It is incredible the amount of weight the single word "cancer" can bring to your life in a moment. I remember taking a deep breath, steeling myself to form the words, "Mom, I have cancer" and then completely breaking as soon as I heard her voice on the other line. I remember feeling strength return when I heard her say, "Ok, I'll call dad and we'll start praying." Prayer. A simple word that Christians throw around casually. We, or at least I did, take for granted the privilege and comfort of talking to God. Those words were enough to ground me, for a little bit anyway, until my spiritual reinforcements could get to me. This was the beginning of a long faith journey for all of us.

Within hours of hearing the news, my dad was on his way to DC to offer physical support at my first appointment with the oncologist. More importantly, he came to build me up in Biblical teaching on healing as shown in miracles throughout the Old and New Testament. We walked into that first appointment, listening and trying to process all the information being thrown at us, yet I was completely at peace. Supernatural peace. The peace that surpasses all understanding [Philippians 4:7]. Even now as I look back, it is hard to comprehend a rational reason for that peace - other than it came direct from God.

The extent of my cancer was still unknown, pending a full PET scan, but the doctor laid out the range of options of least six months of treatment with the possibility of both chemo and radiation, which in her opinion needed to start immediately. She also did her best to gently prepare me that I would lose my hair and struggle through many other side effects from ongoing treatment. Again, I'm not lying when I say that I felt a momentary tightness of fear, only to have it disappear just as quickly and replaced with absolute peace.

We asked the doctor if there was ever a scenario when they stopped mid-treatment. She said it would have to be "fantastical results", to which my dad replied "You mean a miracle?" She just smiled back at us. We were believing for a healing miracle, so now we just needed God to show my doctor.

That night, my dad sat down with me and my roommate and led us through a Bible study. At the end, he asked me what I wanted to believe God for. I verbalized what I believed based on God's truths. I began to write this down in a journal that guided me, my family, and friends, so that we were able to stand together in prayer. It also allowed me to share the faith I was standing on with coworkers and other outside interactions. In truth, the more I said it, the more I believed it, and the more confident I was in what God was doing in and through me. My journal became a combination of prayers, scriptures, and proclamations of what God was already doing in my life because I am his. I keep the index card in my journal as a reminder of God's promise and faithfulness (dated March 2, 2013):

- I am not going to have "bad" days with nausea and low blood counts. I am NOT living in fear.
- I am not going to lose my hair! I know I heard God tell me "not to worry, I got this." So I believe it. Amen!
- I will not lose the joy of the Lord, so that my life may be a living testimony of a faith-filled life. I believe I am going to

minister to the other patients, nursing staff, and the people in my life who do not believe as much or as strongly as I do in what God can do.

- This is going to be a testament to the awesomeness of God! And my medical recovery is going to be credited to divine healing – so God will get the credit, not doctors or medicine.

This sickness is not unto death, but for the glory of God that the Son of God might be glorified thereby.

John 11:4

The following week, my parents swapped places and it was my mom's turn to stand in faith with me. One of the first things she did for me was create a list – my "daily Gospel pills" – of the promises of God regarding abundant life and healing. Reading scripture and applying it to my life built up my armor and defense against the enemy's strategic attacks.

Behold I give you power to tread on serpents and scorpions [demons] and over all the power of the enemy; and nothing shall by any means hurt you. Luke 10:19

That week, we went back to the oncologist to get the results of my PET scan and my doctor pronounced my diagnosis as Stage Three Hodgkin's Lymphoma. The cancer was almost completely centralized in the lymph nodes around my neck, but the PET scan also showed spots on my hip and spleen, which prompted even more tests and possible concerns. On the drive home, my mom and I decided not to discuss my official diagnosis with anyone, so as not to create fear in the people around me. The diagnosis was just a label from the world, not the final word from God, and I did not want any focus to shift from what God was going to do.

The power of life and death are in the power of the tongue. Proverbs 18:21

Of course, that was put to the test days later, when I woke up in extreme pain in my hip. My mom was asleep (or so I thought) in the living room and I didn't want to wake her to see me in that much pain, not when I had been telling everyone how much confidence I had in God. So despite tears and frustrations, I began to pace in my room, crying out to God, and rebuking Satan, demanding that he leave my body and my room. Little did I know that the Holy Spirit had woken my mom at that same time and, while she was unaware of the battle going on in my room, she too was praying and rebuking Satan, even putting her hands on my bedroom door. I am humbled by God's goodness to say that after that night, I never had pain in my hip again and my bone marrow biopsy came back negative. God is good!

The enemy didn't stop there. Days after my first round of chemo, the swelling in my neck had grown and I was admitted to the hospital for the weekend, complete with two blood transfusions, and the news that it was very likely that I would have numerous hospital stays and transfusions throughout the next six months of treatment. Well that didn't seem to line up with God's promise for abundant life, so we prayed against that and I never needed to go back to the hospital.

I don't mean to sound glib or simplistic or even pat myself on the back. I definitely had moments of doubt and self-pity, but whenever I started to sink or misstep, there was a God-ordained intervention by a text message with scripture, or a call from a friend who wanted to pray with me, or even simply hearing a worship song on the radio that ministered to my soul. I know beyond a shadow of a doubt that God was next to me every single step and, when he knew I needed the extra support, he rallied my spiritual reinforcements. Thank God that there were so many people around me that listened to the Spirit's leading and became instruments of his hand.

Several weeks into chemo, I had yet another physical set back. I began to lose my hair, despite knowing with absolute certainty that I had felt God's presence tell me not to worry about it. Honestly, I struggled more with this than any other part of the diagnosis and treatment. Not because I was afraid of what I would look like for vanity's sake, but because I had specifically told people that I was not going to lose my hair. Now people were not going to see healing, but rather another sick girl "trying to stay positive." From the start of this journey, I wanted my life and my healing to be a reflection of God's miraculous power, so he would get all the credit – not the doctors or treatment – and I certainly didn't want to just be another "positive" person. In the weeks to follow, I continued to call out the promises of healing and protection and seek ways to give God glory for my healing.

Over the years, I have come to realize that when I heard God in the doctor's office tell me not to worry, he was not talking about just my hair; but my entire body. He had my life in his hand and none of the "bumps" in the road were going to change the final outcome. So my hair continued to thin out, but I never did lose it all, and when I decided to just shave my head (to clean it up), I was not emotional about it. My identity and joy was intertwined so tightly with God that it didn't matter what I looked like. In fact, several of my friends said it was the only way people could tell I was actually undergoing chemo.

Two months into treatment, I had my second PET scan and we got our "fantastical results"; not a spot of cancer in my body and the scar tissue was already minimizing. Talk about an answer to prayer! Just thinking about that conversation with my doctor gives me chills. Even the doctor had to admit that this was completely unexpected and she was surprised that the chemo would have been able to work that quickly. What an incredible open door I had to share what God had confirmed in black and white. In the end, I continued with the course of treatment, but I made it abundantly clear to my doctor and the nurses, that as far as I was concerned, I did not have any more cancer in my body. So from then on, the majority of my prayers were directed at the chemo, commanding those drugs to target and affect only the bad cells in my body.

> **And these signs will accompany those who believe; in my name they will cast out demons, they shall speak with new tongues; they shall take up serpents [lies of the devil] and if they drink any deadly thing, it shall not hurt them, they shall lay hands on the sick and they shall recover. Mark 16:17–18**

The remaining months of treatment fell into a routine without any major complications that I had been warned about - another praise! My doctor and nurses were continually admitting that despite having cancer, I was "pretty healthy." Toward the last several rounds of treatment, my white cell count fell and my energy was limited due to the chemotherapy, but that season of my life really caused me to stop and prioritize my values. I cut things out in order to spend more time with God on a daily basis and the benefits far outweigh catching up on the latest TV show or movie.

I pushed to have my medi-port removed shortly after my last chemo appointment, despite my doctor's suggestion to keep it for a couple months in case the cancer "came back". To this day, I believe the cancer left my body even before I started treatment and in my mind, keeping that port in my chest a moment longer would have opened me to doubt or fear of getting sick again. Even now, years later, I set my spiritual eyes on God's promises before I head into one of my check-ins, so that the enemy does not gain a foothold.

Oncologist don't like to use the word healing; they prefer to say remission. I have so much respect for those in the medical profession, especially for those in oncology since they see so much defeat every day, and I believe that God has given these men and women knowledge to help alleviate suffering. But we have to remember that what God promises in his word holds far more weight than anything a doctor and paper may say.

For all the promises of God in Christ Jesus are yea and amen unto the glory of God. II Cor. 1:20

Several things stuck out to me that God showed me during this season in my life, which have remained in the forefront of my life to this day. The first is communion. I've been in church my whole life and partaking in the body and blood of Christ on a frequent basis. The emphasis has always been on the blood of Christ, spilled so that we could have eternal life, but we partake in the blood AND the bread (God's body broken so that we could receive healing!). The gift of salvation and healing go hand in hand; they always have and yet we *accept* salvation and *hope* for healing. What a lie from Satan. Healing *IS* God's will for our lives.

The other big thing I learned and held onto is that we need to truly live out what we believe. Faith is only successful when it is followed by action; otherwise, it is just words. You can say anything you want at any time, but if you do not step out and act as though they are true, there is nothing behind those words. Sometimes you have to step into the Jordan River *before* it parts for you walk through (Joshua 3).

Thus also faith by itself, if it does not have works, is dead. James 2:17

Looking back, one of the things that has struck me is *why* did we wait until after a doctor confirmed my diagnosis to start purposefully praying for healing? Why didn't we start to pray when I was feeling sick and tired those first two months? Why do we often wait for big things to happen before calling on God for His help?

Along with my family, I had an amazing group of friends around me. Friends who prayed alongside me and believed with me. It is so important to surround yourself with people who are going to be in agreement with you. They were by my side during setbacks in the first few weeks and they kept things fun (we marked my 29th birthday with BBQ, cake, and shaving my head). They also stood with me in agreement when I rebuked fear, self-pity, and limitations in my body. Trust me, if you ever find yourself weakened by fear, doubt, or a physical illness, surround yourself with spiritual reinforcements.

Time and time again, the enemy tried to discourage my faith and shift my focus onto "me" and how I was feeling, rather than what God had promised. So I continued to submerge myself in God. By shutting out the noise of the world, I was able to hear God more clearly and it is easier to follow his leading when his voice is clear.

Sadly, cancer is so commonplace nowadays. I honestly can't understand how people face it – the treatments, the effects, and changes to your body – without having God in their lives. I am so thankful to know him and to have experienced his great love and mercy. My prayer is that you know it too.

Acknowledgments and
Further References

Bosworth, F.F., *Christ the Healer,* Fleming H. Revell Company, Old Tappan, NJ, 1973.

E.W. Kenyon, *Christ the Healer,* from his Advanced Bible Course, Studies in the Deeper Life, and *Jesus the Healer,* 1940 (available through Amazon)

Dr. T.J. McCrossan, *Bodily Healing and The Atonement,* Kenneth Hagin's Faith Library, Broken Arrow, OK, 1982

T.L. Osborn, *Healing the Sick,* Harrison House Press, Tulsa, OK, 1992

Sumrall, Lester, *Pioneers of Faith,* LESEA Publishing, South Bend, IN, 1995

William Vigue, *Meat of The Word Ministries at Meatoftheword.org*

e-Sword, The Sword of the Lord with an Electronic Edge, Rick Meyers, 2014

About the Authors

Barbara Grace Mariano Vigue was born to Peter Mariano and Mary Tristani Mariano in Bridgeport, CT. All four of her grandparents were Italian immigrants and brought with them to America a rich heritage of traditions and love of family. Both large families were neighbors and friends and within the first years of their immigration to Pennsylvania, they were all introduced to Jesus Christ. They enthusiastically embraced their new country and faith in God. Grandfather Tristani became a minister and started an Italian Christian church in Bridgeport, CT.

Barbara had an idyllic childhood, surrounded by loving, wise parents, her brother and sister, dozens of cousins, aunts, and uncles, as well as her church family. She does not remember a time in her life when she did not love the Lord, but she had so much learning of the word ahead of her. She married her husband Bill, a minister, in 1983 and they have three children who are all serving the Lord. Gabrielle lives and works in Charlotte, NC with the Billy Graham Evangelistic Association. Mary and her husband Chris live in New Milford, CT where they are associate pastors. Mary teaches middle school in a Christian school. They have three children, Emery, Will, and Ben. Michael lives and works in Lakeland, Florida as assistant athletic director at Southeastern University.

Barbara started her career as a registered nurse in Connecticut, but soon focused on starting a church and a Christian school with her husband, where she taught high school and provided counseling as a Licensed Professional Counselor. Keeping her hand in nursing, she continued in psychiatric home care, both in Connecticut and later Florida. Upon retiring from nursing and moving to Zebulon, NC, she continues with her husband in their ministry, Meat of The Word Ministries. Bill has a weekly television program and they are available for speaking engagements. Since childhood, writing has been her favorite pastime and the way she processes her thoughts and leadings from the Lord.

Just like her parents and grandparents before her, love of God and love of family are foremost in her life. Her goal is to faithfully serve our Lord and see his glory revealed on earth as it is in heaven.

Gabrielle Vigue grew up in Brookfield, Connecticut. After college, she had an opportunity to work as Executive Assistant with the New England Patriots outside Boston and then at the Advisory Board Company in Washington DC. Believing God was leading her to use her abilities for the kingdom of God, she now works at the Billy Graham Evangelistic Association. She joyfully serves as Executive Administrative Assistant to the Vice-President of Crusade Ministries in Charlotte, NC. She is grateful for many for many opportunities God has given her to share her journey from cancer to healing. She prays more people would come to know God's great love and healing touch.

Printed in the United States
By Bookmasters